Corneal Topography

Melanie Corbett · Nicholas Maycock
Emanuel Rosen · David O'Brart

Corneal Topography

Principles and Applications

Second Edition

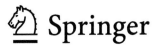 Springer

Melanie Corbett
Imperial College Healthcare NHS Trust
London
UK

Emanuel Rosen
Manchester
UK

Nicholas Maycock
University Hospital Coventry
and Warwickshire
Coventry
UK

David O'Brart
Department of Ophthalmology
St. Thomas Hospital
London
UK

The first edition of the work was published in 1999 by BMJ books with the following title:
Corneal Topography – Principles and Applications.

ISBN 978-3-030-10694-2   ISBN 978-3-030-10696-6   (eBook)
https://doi.org/10.1007/978-3-030-10696-6

Library of Congress Control Number: 2019935125

This Springer imprint is published by the registered company Springer Nature Switzerland AG
The registered company address is: Gewerbestrasse 11, 6330 Cham, Switzerland

Contents

Part III   Corneal Disease

Part IV   Corneal Surgery

Part I

Basic Principles

Assessment of Corneal Shape

The anterior cornea is the major refractive surface of the eye, responsible for over two-thirds of its total dioptric power. Therefore very small changes in corneal shape can have a dramatic effect on the clarity with which an image is focused on the retina. As patients and surgeons strive to optimise the optical outcome of corneal disease and surgery, it has become increasingly important that the shape of the anterior corneal surface can be measured accurately.

Topography is the science of describing or representing the features of a particular place in detail. Over the last four centuries, new techniques for studying corneal topography have been developed in response to continually changing clinical demands.

History of Corneal Topography

With the advent of widespread refractive correction at the beginning of the seventeenth century, interest developed in the shape of the cornea and the optical properties of the eye. Early investigations of corneal topography were confined to gross estimates of corneal curvature (Fig. 1.1).

In 1619, Scheiner made the first measurements of corneal shape [1]. He held up a series of convex mirrors of different curvatures next to the eye, until he found one which gave an image of the same size as the image from the cornea.

In the 1820s, Cuignet developed a keratoscope through which he observed the reflected image of an illuminated target held in front of the patient's cornea. His major problem was in the alignment of the light, target and observer with the patient's visual axis. This was overcome in 1882 by Placido, who placed an observation hole in the centre of the target [2]. His target was a disc bearing alternating black and white concentric rings; and this pattern still forms the basis of many topography systems today.

Quantification of corneal curvature became possible in 1854 with the development of the keratometer (ophthalmometer) by Helmholtz [3]. The distance between

© Springer Nature Switzerland AG 2019
M. Corbett et al., *Corneal Topography*,
https://doi.org/10.1007/978-3-030-10696-6_1

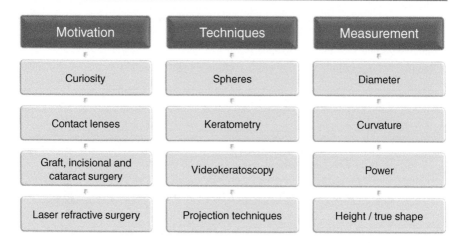

Fig. 1.1 Development of corneal topography. Changing clinical demands have driven the development of new techniques and methods of measurement

two pairs of reflected points gave the spherocylindrical curvature of the central 3 mm of the cornea, in two meridians. In order to increase the area of the cornea analysed, Javal (1889) attached a Placido-type disc to his keratometer. Its telescopic eyepiece gave him the additional benefit of a magnified keratoscopy image. He realised the need to "fix" the image and measure the size of the rings, but this was not practical until Gullstrand (1896) applied photography to keratoscopy (photokeratoscopy). Numerous attempts were made to quantify keratographs by comparison with photographs of spheres of known radius, but all techniques were laborious and time-consuming.

Little progress was then made in corneal topography until the middle of this century, when interest was rekindled by the introduction of contact lenses. Contact lens fitting requires knowledge of the curvature of the midperipheral cornea. The keratometer could provide this information for relatively normal corneas with only regular astigmatism and is still suitable for contact lens fitting in uncomplicated cases today.

With the development of microsurgical techniques for cataract extraction, corneal grafting and incisional refractive surgery, interest turned to the optical power provided by the cornea. Measurements of cornea curvature can be converted to dioptric power using the standard keratometric index.

As the visual results of these procedures have improved, fine-tuning of the refractive outcome has become increasingly important. It became necessary to develop means of assessing the topography of the whole corneal surface with great detail and accuracy. Photokeratoscopy provided qualitative information about a large area of the cornea, but it was only as a result of developments in computing that quantitative analysis of these images could be performed using videokeratoscopy. Several devices were developed based on the principle of projection rather than reflection to generate true height data, but in practice, mainly those using Scheimpflug technology are in general use.

The explosion of refractive surgery has also opened up new avenues for the development of topographic systems such as Scheimpflug camera-based systems, which permit a detailed examination of the anterior and posterior corneal surface as well as other anterior chamber parameters (see Chap. 4) [4, 5].

An understanding of how corneal topography has developed so far helps to explain the nature of current topography systems today [6–8] and sets the scene for how further progress may occur in the future.

Description of Corneal Shape

There are several ways in which the shape of the cornea can be measured and represented [9–12]. Each has its own advantages, and the use of the most appropriate method for a given clinical situation can enhance the presentation and interpretation of results. Examples using these methods are given throughout the book.

Corneal Height or Elevation

The fundamental way of describing any surface mathematically is to define the distance of each of its points from a reference plane. On a geographical map, the surface of the land is expressed as "height above sea level". For the cornea there is no standard position for the reference plane, so this is usually set arbitrarily at the corneal apex or a level near the limbus. The actual position of the reference plane used is of no importance because it does not affect the relative positions of points on the surface.

Data measured in terms of height or elevation (or sometimes depth) from a reference plane describes the true shape of the corneal surface. This is particularly valuable in corneal disease and in excimer laser surgery where the outcome is determined by the depth of tissue removed and replaced. Once the true shape has been measured, slope, curvature and power can be calculated from it (Fig. 1.2c).

Surface Slope

The slope of a curved surface is the gradient of the tangent at a particular point (Fig. 1.2d). Mathematically, the slope is the first differential of a curve. Therefore it is a more sensitive way of demonstrating small changes in height between two points on a surface.

Radius of Curvature

For the cornea, an alternative way of expressing slope is as radius of curvature (Fig. 1.2e). Slope (α) can be converted to radius of curvature (r) by the equation:

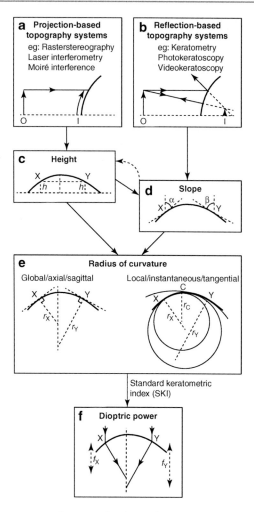

Fig. 1.2 Data measurement and presentation by various corneal topography systems. This is shown for two points X and Y, which lie at the same height on opposite semimeridians of an asymmetric cornea (such as keratoconus). In projection-based systems (**a**), an object (o) is projected onto the surface of the cornea to produce an image (I), from which the true shape of the cornea can be measured in terms of height (*h*) or elevation, above a reference plane (**c**). These data can then be used to calculate surface slope, curvature and power. Reflection-based systems (**b**) view the first Purkinje image formed behind the cornea and calculate the slope (at angles α and β) of the corneal surface (**d**) and then the curvature and power. Slope cannot be converted to height without additional measurements and certain assumptions being made. Radius of curvature (**e**) can be calculated either globally or locally. Global or axial radius of curvature is the perpendicular distance (*r*) from the tangent at a point to the visual axis. The accuracy of these measurements decreases in the periphery. The local or tangential radius of curvature applies to the sphere that best fits the shape of a small area surrounding each point. Accuracy is better maintained from the centre (point C) to the periphery (points X and Y). Radius of curvature can be converted to dioptric power using the standard keratometric index, but this makes a number of assumptions. Dioptric power (**f**) is a measure of the cornea's ability to refract light by acting as a convex lens of focal length f (power is inversely proportional to focal length)

Fig. 1.3 Corneal slope and radius of curvature. A point on the corneal surface is located at distance d from the axis. The corneal slope at this point is at angle α, and the line perpendicular to it is normal. The radius of curvature (*r*) is the distance along the normal from the corneal surface to its intersection with the axis, which is given by *d*/cos α. This is the global/axial/sagittal radius of curvature (Fig. 1.2e)

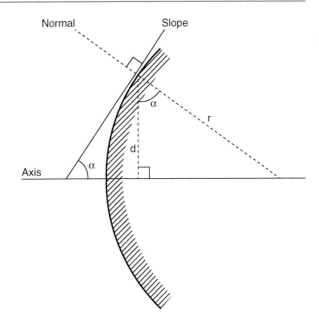

$$r = d / \cos\alpha$$

where *d* is the distance from the corneal centre (cos 0° = 0; cos 60° = 0.5; cos 90° = 1) (Fig. 1.3). Corneas with a steep surface slope have a small radius of curvature, whereas those which are flatter have a relatively large radius of curvature. This format is particularly useful for certain applications, such as contact lens fitting.

Radius of curvature can be calculated by two means: global (axial, sagittal) radius of curvature was used initially, but more recently local (instantaneous, tangential) radius of curvature has been found to be more appropriate in some situations [13, 14]. Each type of measurement of radius of curvature can be converted to the equivalent type of power measurement (i.e. global power or local power), with similar advantages and disadvantages [15, 16].

Global (Axial/Sagittal) Radius of Curvature

Global radius of curvature calculates the curvature of the cornea radially at points along each of the meridians. It measures the perpendicular distance from the tangent at a point to the optical axis. These algorithms have a spherical bias because each measurement is related to the optical axis.

Local (Instantaneous/Tangential) Radius of Curvature

Local radius of curvature calculates the curvature at each point with respect to its neighbouring points, by fitting the best-fit sphere. Results have less spherical bias because curvature is calculated for individual small groups of points without reference to the visual axis or the overall shape of the cornea. Therefore there is greater accuracy in the periphery of the cornea and better representation of local irregularities [13].

Corneal Power

Power is a measure of the refractive effect of a lens. For optical lenses, measurements of radius of curvature (r, in metres) can be converted to power (P, in dioptres) (Fig. 1.2f) using the formula:

$$P = \left(n_2 - n_1 \right) / r$$

where n_1 is the refractive index of the first medium (in the case of the anterior corneal surface, air = 1) and n_2 is the refractive index of the second medium (in this case, cornea = 1.376). The same formula would also apply to the posterior corneal surface. However, the curvature of the posterior corneal surface is not easy to measure [17, 18]. Therefore, the standard keratometric index (SKI = 1.3375) is an approximation used in the conversion from curvature to power, to take account of both surfaces of the cornea [19, 20]. However, if the cornea is unusually thick or thin, estimates of its posterior curvature are poor [21]. Additional inaccuracies are derived from the fact that the exact refractive indices of the cornea and its constituent layers are unknown [22]. Therefore, for corneal topography, using the SKI:

$$P = 0.3375 / r$$

but it must be remembered that the radius of curvature in this equation is expressed in metres. Curvatures given in millimetres must be divided by 1000 before being entered in the equation. Therefore this becomes:

$$P \left(\text{in diopteres} \right) = 337.5 / R \left(\text{in mm} \right).$$

Corneal power is a useful way of representing the refractive effect of the cornea in patients undergoing corneal or refractive surgery. However, it is the least accurate way of describing corneal shape due to the assumptions made during its derivation (Table 1.1) [21–25]. Therefore, when maximum accuracy is required, for example, when calculating the power of an intraocular lens, radius of curvature should be used.

Table 1.1 Inaccuracies generated by the conversion of radius of curvature to power

Assumptions made in converting radius of curvature to power	Effects
Conversion formula assumes spherical optics	Inaccurate outside the central cornea
SKI assumes the curvature of the posterior cornea to be normal	Inaccurate for very steep or very flat corneas (e.g. high myopia or high hyperopia)
SKI assumes the cornea to be of normal thickness	Inaccurate following excimer laser photorefractive keratectomy or epikeratophakia
SKI assumes that the refractive index of the cornea is uniform and fails to recognise the differing refractive properties of the epithelium and stroma	Inaccurate in certain situations, such as following refractive surgery

SKI standard keratometric index

Methods of Measurement

Methods for measuring corneal topography fall into two broad categories: those which use the principle of reflection and those which use the principle of projection (Chap. 3). The two techniques differ in the measurements they make.

Reflection-Based Methods

Many topography systems in clinical use today are based on the principle of reflection (Chap. 2). Examples include the Placido ring, keratometer and videokeratoscopes (see Chap. 2). They measure the slope of the corneal surface and can use this information to calculate radius of curvature and power (Fig. 1.2b). However, corneal elevation cannot be calculated from measurements of slope alone. The slope provides information about the gradient of a particular point at location (x, y), but it does not determine the elevation of that point in the z-axis. Therefore true corneal shape cannot be reconstructed from measurements obtained by reflection alone, without making many assumptions [26–28].

Projection-Based Methods

Many of the topography systems in clinical use today are based on the principle of projection. Examples include devices utilising the Scheimpflug principle, slit photography, rastersterography, moiré interference and laser interferometry (Chaps. 3 and 4). They directly measure true corneal shape in terms of elevation, from which slope, curvature and power can be calculated (Fig. 1.2a) [29, 30].

Applications of Corneal Topography

Corneal topography has applications in both clinical practice and research. It is noninvasive and easy to perform, and therefore measurements can be obtained in almost any patient. However, when such a technique is used in clinical practice, it is important to be more critical of the benefits it provides for the patient, the costs involved, and whether more suitable alternatives are available [31, 32]. When deciding whether to perform an investigation, the clinician must consider whether the results are likely to improve patient management.

Table 1.2 outlines when corneal topography is valuable in clinical practice and distinguishes the situations when other examination techniques are sufficient [33]. It also provides examples of the many ways in which corneal topography can assist research. Each of these applications is described and illustrated in *later chapters*.

The Normal Cornea and Corneal Disease

Corneal topography has been used to quantify the shape of the normal cornea and improve our understanding of the relationships between anatomy and visual

Table 1.2 Indications for corneal topography in clinical practice and research

Situation	Other techniques sufficient, e.g. keratometry, refraction, slit lamp	Clinical indications for corneal topography	Examples of use of topography in research
Normal cornea		Screening	Determine shape
			Correlate visual function
Contact lenses	Fitting in simple cases	Fitting in complex cases	Effect of lenses on the cornea
		Detection of warpage	
Corneal disease	Routine diagnosis	Monitoring	Optical effects
	Routine follow-up	Effect on visual function	
		Subclinical detection	
		Genetic screening	
Cataract surgery	*Simple cases*	*Complex cases*	Quantification for clinical trials
	Planning incision	Planning incision	Incision architecture
	IOL calculation	IOL calculation	Factors determining outcome
	Suture removal	Suture removal	
		Investigation of poor outcome	
Corneal graft surgery	Routine follow-up	Assessment of regularity	Quantification for clinical trials
		Suture removal	Factors determining outcome
		Contact lens fitting	
Refractive surgery	Routine follow-up	Preoperative screening	Quantification for clinical trials
		Planning incisions	Understand side effects
		Documentation of surgery performed	Optical quality postoperatively
		Investigation of poor outcome	Monitor healing
		Discussion with patients	

function (Chap. 6). The technique is sufficiently sensitive to diagnose corneal shape anomalies, such as keratoconus, at an early stage [34]. This is helpful in the management and treatment of patients, the identification of affected family members for genetic studies, and in screening prior to refractive surgery. Corneal disease processes can be monitored by comparison of serial measurements, and their effects on vision can be better understood (Chaps. 8, 9 and 10).

Contact Lens Fitting

Contact lens fitting can adequately be performed using keratometry in the majority of patients, but in complex cases a knowledge of the shape of the whole cornea is useful. Detailed analysis of corneal topography in contact lens wearers has correlated corneal warpage patterns with the resting position of a hard lens and has demonstrated that warpage resolution times can be far longer than previously expected (Chap. 7).

Corneal and Refractive Surgery

An important role for corneal topography is in the expanding field of corneal, cataract and laser refractive surgery (Chaps. 12, 13 and 14). Preoperatively, knowledge of the topography of an individual cornea is of benefit when planning incisional surgery and can also be used to calculate the power of intraocular lens required in cataract surgery. Postoperatively, detailed information about the outcome of any refractive procedure can be quantified for clinical trials, for example, the optical quality and centration of the correction and its long-term stability. Corneal topography may explain unexpected results, by demonstrating a multifocal central corneal contour following radial keratotomy or a decentred treatment zone after LASIK, LASEK and PRK. It can help our understanding of side effects and guide the manipulation or removal of sutures after corneal surgery. Colour-coded maps are also a useful aid when discussing with patients their surgical procedures or postoperative outcome.

Suitability of Topography Systems

When any measuring equipment is under development, there is a tendency to strive to maximise the quantity, accuracy and complexity of the information it provides. This is ideal for those systems which are to be used primarily for research. However, in clinical practice, the resulting increase in size, expense and examination times may be unacceptable.

When a clinical department wants to purchase a corneal topography system, it must first consider how it will be used. It must also evaluate the benefits and cost of a new system over those it already possesses (such as slit lamp examination, refraction and keratometry) [6, 7]. Likewise, those developing topography systems need to consider what is required and how it can best be provided.

Not all applications of topography have the same requirements, so should different types of systems be developed, or should all systems be adequate for all applications? Different groups of operators may also vary in their requirements, depending on their case mix and aims of treatment. The needs of technicians, optometrists, corneal physicians and refractive surgeons will be different. Therefore each individual operator has to consider what they want from corneal topography.

Table 1.3 outlines some of the variables which relate to the situation in which measurements are made, the nature of the cornea, the types of measurement and the use of the information obtained. It also lists the different options which topography systems can provide to meet the variety of requirements.

Table 1.3 Suitability of topography systems

Considerations	Variables	Options
Situation	Patient cooperation	Need for fixation target or not
	Outreach clinics	Slit lamp-mounted
	Intraoperative	Microscope-mounted
	Speed of operation	Portable
		Real-time information
Cornea	Area	Reflection- or projection-based systems
	Irregularity	Cornea only or including limbus
	Reflectivity	
	Range of curvatures	
Measurements	Type of data	Height, slope, curvature or power
	Location of most data points	Central weighting or uniform distribution
	Number of data points	Short or lengthy processing
	Accuracy and reproducibility	Clinical or research
Presentation and use	Display to patient, clinician or meetings	2D or 3D colour maps
	Single or multiple patients	Statistical indices
	Preoperative assessment	Surgical nomograms
	Integration in to surgical equipment or lasers	Neural networks
		Tailor-made software

The most appropriate style of topography machine depends upon the nature of the situations and the corneas to which it will be applied, the type of measurements required and how the results will be used

Situation

Most topography systems available commercially today are relatively large machines and require the patient to sit at a slit lamp and fixate a target. The portable systems now appearing on the market can be used in debilitated patients, at the extremes of age and in outreach clinics [29]. Videokeratoscopes depend upon accurate fixation by the patient, but in projection-based systems, this is less important.

Hand-held keratoscopes can be used during surgery, but most are not computerised [36]. Ideally, intraoperative topography requires real-time analysis, so the effect of each manoeuvre on corneal shape can be seen as it happens [37]. This will require data processing to occur almost instantaneously.

Cornea

Some systems can measure relatively normal corneas very accurately, whereas others are better at imaging irregular corneas. Devices with relatively few data points (e.g. keratometry) or those that make assumptions based on normal data (e.g. Scheimpflug) are best used on relatively normal corneas [38, 39]. However, projection-based systems making more direct measurements from multiple corneal points can be used accurately for both regular and irregular corneas. Systems where the original image can be viewed (e.g. videokeratoscopes) enable the operator to assess the quality of the data provided. The peripheral cornea is also better assessed by projection-based techniques that do not rely upon the optical axis for their calculations [39].

Measurements

Different applications require different information. Measurements of corneal height can only be made using a projection-based system, whereas curvature and power can be provided by any system.

The accuracy and reproducibility of the measurements are partly dependent upon the number of data points and the sophistication of the machine [40]. However, the accuracy required in clinical practice is usually only just higher than that which is clinically detectable. If the number of data points can be reduced, the speed of image processing improves. The most efficient distribution of data points to provide information about the optical effect of the cornea is with the majority of points within the pupillary aperture.

Presentation and Use

Coloured maps are a helpful means of presenting the results of individual patients. If individual maps are summarised by mathematical indices, grouped data is then amenable to statistical analysis. Numerous mathematical indices could be devised, and consideration needs to be given as to which are most useful.

It is becoming possible for topography systems to contain artificial neural networks which can recognise topography patterns and objectively classify maps. Software is being developed to integrate topographic information with surgical equipment. In the future these will be used to control lasers for the treatment of irregular astigmatism.

As topography equipment becomes more and more sophisticated to serve research and specialist surgery, there is an increasing need for the parallel production of smaller, cheaper devices which are suitable for use in general clinics.

References

*References Particularly Worth Reading

1. Scheiner C. Occulus Hoc est: fundamentum opticum. Innsbruck: Agricola; 1619.
2. Placido A. Novo instrumento de esploracao da cornea. Periodico d'Ofthalmologica Practica Lisbon. 1880;5:27–30.
3. von Helmholtz H. Graefes Arch Ophthalmol. 1854;2:3.

4. Ambrosio R Jr, Belin MW. Imaging of the cornea: topography vs tomography. J Refract Surg. 2010;26:847–9.
5. Belin MW, Khachikian SS. An introduction to understanding elevation-based topography: how elevation data are displayed – a review. Clin Exp Ophthal. 2009;37:14–29.
6. Klyce SD, Wilson SE, Kaufman HE. Corneal topography comes of age [editorial]. Refract Corneal Surg. 1989;5:359–61.
7. Wilson SE, Klyce SD. Advances in the analysis of corneal topography. Surv Ophthalmol. 1991;35:269–77.
8. Morrow GL, Stein RM. Evaluation of corneal topography: past, present and future trends. Can J Ophthalmol. 1992;27:213–25.
9. *Roberts C. Corneal topography: a review of terms and concepts. J Cataract Refract Surg. 1996;22:624–629.
10. *Waring GO. Making sense of keratospeak II: proposed conventional terminology for corneal topography. Refract Corneal Surg. 1989;5:362–367.
11. Klyce SD, Wilson SE. Methods of analysis of corneal topography. Refract Corneal Surg. 1989;5:368–71.
12. Piñero D, Alio JL, Aleson A, Vergara ME, Miranda M. Corneal volume, pachymetry, and correlation of anterior and posterior corneal shape in subclinical and different stages of clinical keratoconus. J Cataract Refract Surg. 2010;36(5):814–25.
13. Roberts C. Characterisation of the inherent error in a spherically-biased corneal topography system in mapping a radially aspheric surface. J Refract Corneal Surg. 1994;10:103–11.
14. Klein SA, Mandell RB. Axial and instantaneous power conversion in corneal topography. Invest Ophthalmol Vis Sci. 1995;36:2155–9.
15. Klein SA, Mandell RB. Shape and refractive powers in corneal topography. Invest Ophthalmol Vis Sci. 1995;36:2096–109.
16. Cohen KL, Tripoli NK, Holmgren DE, Coggins JM. Assessment of the power and height of radial aspheres reported by computer-assisted keratoscopy. Am J Ophthalmol. 1995;119:723–32.
17. Eryildirim A, Ozkan T, Eryildirim S, Kaynak S, Cingil G. Improving estimation of corneal refractive power by measuring the posterior curvature of the cornea. J Cataract Refract Surg. 1994;20:129–31.
18. Patel S, Marshall J, Fitzke FW. Shape and radius of posterior corneal surface. Refract Corneal Surg. 1993;9:173–81.
19. Gullstrand A. (1911). In: Southall JPC, editor. Helmholtz's treatise in physiological optics volumes I and II (Appendix). New York: Dover; 1962.
20. Use of the keratometer. In: Bennett AG, editors. Optics of contact lenses. London: ADO publishing; 1974.
21. Arffa RC, Klyce SD, Busin M. Keratometry in epikeratophakia. J Refract Surg. 1989;2:61–4.
22. Patel S. Refractive index of the mammalian cornea and its influence on pachymetry. Ophthalmic Physiol Opt. 1980;7:503–6.
23. Roberts C. The accuracy of 'power' maps to display curvature data in corneal topography. Invest Ophthalmol Vis Sci. 1994;35:3525–32.
24. *Mandell RB. Corneal power correction factor for photorefractive keratectomy. J Cataract Refract Surg 1994;10:125–128.
25. Corbett MC, Verma S, Prydal JI, Pande M, Oliver KM, Patel S, Marshall J. The contribution of the corneal epithelium to the refractive changes occurring after excimer laser photorefractive keratectomy. Invest Ophthalmol Vis Sci. 1995;36:S2.
26. Applegate RA, Nuñez R, Buettner J, Howland HC. How accurately can videokeratoscophic systems measure surface elevation? Optom Vis Sci. 1995;72:785–92.
27. Tripoli NK, Cohen KL, Holmgren DE, Coggins JM. Assessment of radial aspheres by the arc-step algorithm as implemented by the Keratron keratoscope. Am J Ophthalmol. 1995;120:658–64.
28. Tripoli NK, Cohen KL, Obla P, Coggins JM, Holmgren DE. Height measurement of astigmatic test surfaces by a keratoscope that uses plane geometry surface reconstruction. Am J Ophthalmol. 1996;121:668–76.

29. Swartz T, Marten L, Wang M. Measuring the cornea: the latest developments in corneal topography. Curr Opin Ophthalmol. 2007;18(4):325–33.
30. Oliveira CM, Ribeiro C, Franco S. Corneal imaging with slit-scanning and Scheimpflug imaging techniques. Clin Exp Optom. 2011;94(1):33–42.
31. Corbett MC, Shilling JS, Holder GE. The assessment of clinical investigations: the Greenwich grading system and its application to electrodiagnostic testing in ophthalmology. Eye. 1995;9(Suppl):59–64.
32. Thornton SP. Clinical evaluation of corneal topography. J Cataract Refract Surg. 1993;19(Suppl):198–202.
33. McDonnell PJ. Current applications of the corneal modeling system. Refract Corneal Surg. 1991;7:87–91.
34. Piñero DP, Nieto JC, Lopez-Miguel A. Characterization of corneal structure in keratoconus. J Cataract Refract Surg. 2012;38(12):2167–83.
35. Corbett MC, Shun-Shin GA, Awdry PN. Keratometry using the Goldmann tonometer. Eye. 1993;7:43–6.
36. Zabel RW, Tuft SJ, Fitzke FW, Marshall J. Corneal topography: a new photokeratoscope. Eye. 1989;3:298–301.
37. Ediger MN, Pettit GH, Weiblinger RP. Noninvasive monitoring of excimer laser ablation by time-resolved reflectometry. Refract Corneal Surg. 1993;9:268–75.
38. Wegener A, Laser-Junga H. Photography of the anterior eye segment according to Scheimpflug's principle: options and limitations – a review. Clin Exp Ophthalmol. 2009;37(1):144–54.
39. Read SA, Collins MJ, Carney LG, et al. The topography of the central and peripheral cornea. IOVS. 2006;47:1404–15.
40. Sunderraj P. Clinical comparison of automated and manual keratometry in pre-operative ocular biometry. Eye. 1992;6:60–2.

Videokeratoscopes

2

The first techniques in widespread clinical use for measuring corneal topography were keratometry and then more recently photokeratoscopy and videokeratoscopy. All these systems rely upon the principle of reflection and use the tear film on the anterior corneal surface as a convex mirror.

These systems have largely been superseded in terms of accuracy by the development of projection-based (Chap. 3) or Scheimpflug camera-based systems (Chap. 4). They are included here so that the principles may be explained and discussed.

Optics of Convex Mirrors

The image formed by a convex mirror can be constructed using two rays: a ray parallel to the principal axis which is reflected away from the principal focus and a ray from the top of the object passing towards the centre of curvature then back along its own path (Fig. 2.1).

The magnification produced by a curved mirror is the ratio of the image size (I) to the object size (O), and this is in turn proportional to the ratio of the distances of the image (v) and the object (u) from the mirror:

$$\text{Magnification} = \frac{I}{O} = \frac{v}{u}$$

In practice, the image (I) is located very close to the focal point (F), which is halfway between the centre of curvature of the mirror (C, at the principal focus) and the mirror itself. Therefore v may be taken to be equal to half the radius of curvature of the mirror ($r/2$). Substituting:

$$I = O \times \frac{r}{2u}$$

M. Corbett et al., *Corneal Topography*,
https://doi.org/10.1007/978-3-030-10696-6_2

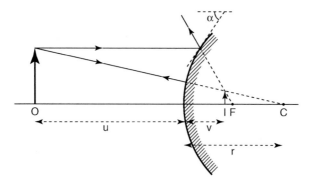

Fig. 2.1 Image formation by a convex mirror. Keratometry and keratoscopy utilise the property of the anterior corneal surface to reflect light, forming a virtual erect image within the anterior chamber. (O = object, I = image, F = focal point, C = centre of curvature of the cornea, u = distance of object from cornea, v = distance of image from cornea, r = radius of curvature of the cornea)

It can therefore be seen that as the cornea becomes steeper and its radius of curvature (r) becomes less, the image (I) also becomes smaller, and the topography mires appear closer together.

In all keratometers, u is constant, being the focal distance of the viewing telescope. Rearrangement of the equation:

$$r = 2u \times \frac{I}{O}$$

shows that the radius of curvature is proportional to the image size if the object size remains constant (von Helmholtz keratometer) or is inversely proportional to the object size if this is varied to achieve a standard image size (Javal-Schiøtz keratometer).

Reflection from the Cornea

Reflection from the anterior wall of the eye occurs at the air-tear fluid interface as opposed to the anterior surface of the cornea. This is not clinically important in the majority of patients, as this is the site of greatest refraction of light rays. However, it may need to be considered in cases of abnormal tear film thickness or marked corneal irregularity. These systems based purely on reflection from the anterior corneal surface have the advantage over Scheimpflug systems (Chap. 4) that data is not degraded by opacities that are purely within the corneal stroma [1].

A light (mire) shone towards the cornea gives rise to a virtual erect image located approximately 4.0 mm posterior to the anterior surface of the cornea, at the level of the anterior lens capsule. This is the corneal light reflex, or first Purkinje image, which is viewed during keratometry and keratoscopy. The size of this image can be used to quantify the curvature of the cornea: the steeper the cornea (small radius of curvature), the more powerful a convex mirror it is, and the smaller the image will be. By the same principles, any toricity (different radii of curvature in different meridia) or irregularity of the corneal surface will cause distortion of the image.

Analysis of a reflected image measures the slope of the corneal surface (marked α in Fig. 2.1). However, no information is provided about the distance of that slope from where it is being viewed (i.e. its position in the z-axis). Therefore the corneal height (or elevation) cannot be measured directly.

Two further steps are required if corneal height is to be estimated. Firstly, additional measurements must be made, such as the height of the corneal apex above a reference plane. Some videokeratoscopes do this using a side camera which views the vertical profile of the cornea. Secondly, it must be assumed that the corneal surface is a continuous curve with no steps. The arc step method works radially from the centre to the periphery. It assumes that the slope at one point remains constant over the intervening cornea, until the next point is reached. Using these assumptions a reasonable estimate of true corneal shape can be made in normal corneas. However, in abnormal or irregular corneas, projection-based techniques are required.

Keratometry

The keratometer measures the distance between the images of two perpendicular pairs of points reflected from a 3 mm annulus of paracentral cornea [1–3].

Table 2.1 Comparison of three corneal topography instruments dependent upon reflection

Instruments	Keratometer	Photokeratoscope	Computerised videokeratoscope
Examples	Helmholtz, Javal-Schiøtz	Corneoscope	TMS, EyeSys
No. of points	4	Many	6000–11,000
Area	Annulus of 3 mm radius	70% of surface	95% of surface 9–11 mm diameter
Dioptric range	30–60D	Infinite	8–110D
Focusing	Superimposition/ alignment of two mires (easy)	Subjective focusing of single image (difficult)	Overlap laser spots or cross hairs (easy)
Mires	Four objects	12 rings	15–38 rings
Record	Two numbers	Still photography	Stills from video
Method	Measurement	Observation	Computer analysis
Topographic information	None	Qualitative	Quantitative
Accuracy	Excellent (for spheres)	Poor	Good
Sensitivity	Moderate	Low (3DC)	0.25D or better
Reproducibility	Excellent	Moderate	Good (0.50D)

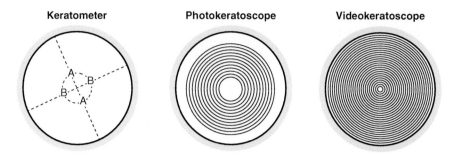

Keratometer   Photokeratoscope   Videokeratoscope

Fig. 2.2 Mires. Representation of the corneal area covered by the mires of the keratometer (two perpendicular pairs of mires, A and B situated on the annulus approximately 3 mm in diameter), photokeratoscope (12 rings) and computer-assisted videokeratoscope (25 rings)

Fig. 2.3 Keratometer. The keratometer uses the reflection of the orange and green mires to measure the curvature of a 3 mm corneal annulus in two perpendicular meridians

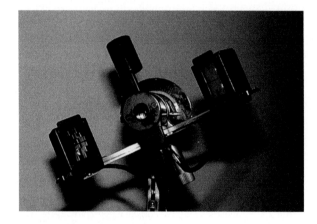

It only measures the curvature of the central cornea (Table 2.1) because the mires are reflected from an annulus 2.6–3.7 mm in diameter, centred on the corneal apex (Fig. 2.2). A pair of mires is first positioned in the steepest meridian and then at 90° to it (Fig. 2.3). Therefore the surface curvature can only be expressed in terms of a sphere and uniform cylinder (Table 2.2). In contrast, videokeratoscopes can measure corneal curvature in more detail and over a much greater area (Figs. 2.4 and 2.5).

Keratometry measurements are highly accurate and reproducible for regular spherocylindrical surfaces such as the paracentral area of the normal cornea [4]. The equipment is relatively inexpensive, and it is used in the fitting of contact lenses, calculation of the power of intraocular lenses [5–7] and identification of tight corneal sutures for removal [8].

However, they are of only limited value for irregular corneas because the mire reflections may be distorted and no information is provided about the corneal curvature inside, outside or between the four reference points [9, 10]. Insufficient information is provided for the management of complex cases or patients undergoing refractive surgery (Table 2.3).

Table 2.2 Assumptions made by the keratometer (K), photokeratoscope (P) and computer-assisted videokeratoscope (V)

Assumptions	K	P	V
Corneal surface is spherocylindrical	+		
Corneal surface is locally spherical			+
Major and minor axes separated by 90°	+		
Cornea is of uniform refractive index	+		+
Neglects corneal thickness	+	+	+
Neglects corneal position after refractive surgery	+	+	+
Correct corneal position and orientation	+	+	+
Light arising from one meridian on a particular mire falls on the same meridian at the film plane		+	+
Centres of curvature for all reflecting points are on the optical axis			+

+ = assumption made for that particular instrument

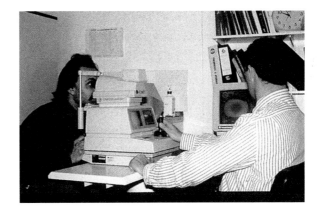

Fig. 2.4 Videokeratoscope. The patient places his or her chin and forehead on the rest and fixates the central target, whilst the operator aligns the machine with the corneal reflex

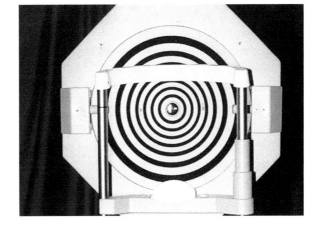

Fig. 2.5 Videokeratoscopy mires. The light cone of videokeratoscopes generates Placido-type mires

Table 2.3 Limitations of the keratometer (K), photokeratoscope (P) and computer-assisted video-keratoscope (V)

Limitations	K	P	V
Examines air-tear film interface, not corneal surface	+	+	+
No direct measurement of central cornea	++	++	
No direct measurement of peripheral cornea	++	+	
Reduced sensitivity in peripheral cornea	–	–	+
Very steep and very flat corneas			+
Irregular corneas	++		+
Complex corneal changes	++	+	
Assumptions of algorithms may not be valid	+		++
Subjective interpretation of displayed data		++	+

+ = moderate limitation, ++ = severe limitation, – = not applicable

Photokeratoscopy

The benefits of photokeratoscopy over keratometry include the qualitative analysis of a larger area of cornea and its use when the mires are distorted by surface irregularities [11].

The mires most commonly take the form of Placido-type concentric rings (Figs. 2.2 and 2.5), but arcs, parallel lines, interference fringes, steps and grids can also be used. By convention the rings are numbered from the innermost to the outermost, but it is important to state the diameter of a given ring as this can vary between instruments. The images are recorded photographically (Table 2.1).

Observation of the spacing and distortion of the rings gives a qualitative analysis of the corneal topography. In areas of steep cornea, the images of the mires are smaller, so the rings appear narrower and closer together. In the presence of regular astigmatism, the mires appear elliptical, with the short axis of the ellipse corresponding to the meridian of corneal steepening and highest power. Irregular astigmatism produces non-elliptical distortion of the mires (Fig. 2.6).

Keratoscopes have been used during large incision cataract surgery and corneal graft surgery with the aim of reducing postoperative astigmatism [2, 12] but were found to be of limited value as they cannot detect less than 3DC and the corneal shape attained at the end of surgery was not necessarily stable postoperatively. Poor sensitivity can also occur in corneal disease, when the mires may look fairly regular despite the presence of clinically significant topographic alterations. Furthermore, the mires do not cover the central cornea, so information is limited in the most visually important area (Table 2.3). Keratoscopy may be of some use in the evaluation of advanced keratoconus, high astigmatism and moderate irregularity, or the adjustment of sutures; but most situations require a more sensitive, quantitative technique (Table 2.4).

Fig. 2.6 Distorted mires. The videokeratoscopy mires are distorted superiorly due to an old paracentral corneal ulcer causing irregular astigmatism

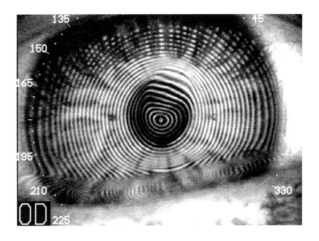

Table 2.4 Advantages of the keratometer (K), photokeratoscope (P) and computer-assisted videokeratoscope (V)

Advantages	K	P	V
Routine clinical applications	+		+
Management of complex corneal cases		?	++
Research tool	+		++
Hard record for audit and litigation purposes	+	+	++
Serial analysis	++		++
Good correlation with visual potential			+
Affordability	++	+	+

? = value not determined, + = moderate advantage, ++ = major advantage

Computer-Assisted Videokeratoscopy

In videokeratoscopy, the image of the mires is captured on a video frame, digitised and then analysed by computer [7, 13–16]. This provides detailed quantitative information about corneal contour. The main advantages of these systems over keratoscopy are their ability to make measurements from the central cornea (Fig. 2.2) and to display the data in a useful format with reasonable accuracy.

There are a variety of systems on the market, all of which have similar benefits and limitations. However, they differ slightly in their ease of use, format of data presentation and extra features they provide.

The accuracy [17–29] of any particular instrument is dependent upon the resolution it achieves at each of the stages between the generation of the mire pattern and the display of the data (Table 2.5). The final transverse spatial resolution should ideally be sufficient to detect surface irregularities just large enough to degrade visual function. This precise level has still to be determined and may vary from the centre to the periphery of the cornea.

Table 2.5 Steps in the
acquisition and analysis of
videokeratoscopy informa-
tion. The accuracy of the
information provided is
dependent upon the accuracy
and resolution achieved
during each of these steps

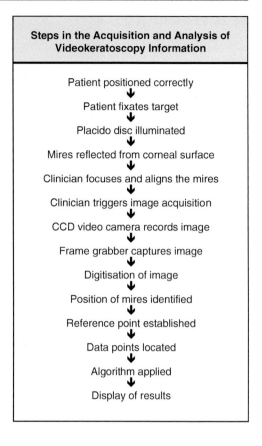

**Steps in the Acquisition and Analysis of
Videokeratoscopy Information**

Patient positioned correctly
⬇
Patient fixates target
⬇
Placido disc illuminated
⬇
Mires reflected from corneal surface
⬇
Clinician focuses and aligns the mires
⬇
Clinician triggers image acquisition
⬇
CCD video camera records image
⬇
Frame grabber captures image
⬇
Digitisation of image
⬇
Position of mires identified
⬇
Reference point established
⬇
Data points located
⬇
Algorithm applied
⬇
Display of results

Hardware

Cone of Mires

The majority of videokeratoscopes use an illuminated cone of Placido-type mires
consisting of concentric rings (Figs. 2.2 and 2.4). Some systems detect the centres
of 30–40 narrow rings, whilst others detect the inner and outer borders of half as
many wider rings. Most systems use alternating black and white rings to maximise
contrast, whilst others in the past used rings of different colours, claiming to overcome the difficulty of imaging irregular corneas when adjacent rings otherwise
become merged.

The mires of most systems cover the cornea over a diameter of about 11 mm.
This excludes the very central cornea (diameter 0.3 mm) and the perilimbal area
(1 mm). This is in contrast to Scheimpflug systems (Chap. 4) which include data
from the very central cornea. However, Placido systems are more accurate in the
area between 3 and 6 mm from the corneal centre [30].

In videokeratoscopes with a long working distance between the cone and the cornea, shadows from the nose or brow may obscure part of the mire pattern (Fig. 2.5). However, this disadvantage is partially offset by the smaller error produced by a given misalignment of the cone relative to the cornea. Systems with highly curved cones close to the eye can obtain information from further in the corneal periphery, particularly for steeper corneas (Fig. 2.4).

In the centre of the mire, pattern is a small light, sometimes coloured or flashing, which the patient must fixate.

Alignment and Focusing

Alignment is the appropriate positioning of the cone relative to the cornea in the x- and y-axes. Focusing is the appropriate positioning in the z-axis. For videokeratoscopes, both are more critical than for projection-based topography systems [31, 32]. Older systems rely upon purely manual alignment and focusing, aided by the superimposition of laser spots or cross hairs. Newer systems have auto-alignment and autofocus mechanisms which fine-tune the manual positioning, with the aim of improving reliability [33].

Image Capture

A charge-coupled device (CCD) video camera is housed behind the aperture in the centre of the cone. When triggered by the clinician, it records an image of the reflected mires on a single frame.

Software

Digitisation

The single video image is stored by the frame grabber and is then digitised. A video image contains 500 lines/frame. A pixel-by-pixel analysis would provide an accuracy of 1.20D. However, by performing automated digitisation with electronic detection of the mires, statistical procedures can achieve subpixel resolution and an accuracy of less than 0.25D.

Image Analysis

First a reference point is established, from which the position of each point can be mathematically identified. Most systems use the centre of the innermost mire or the reflection of the fixation light. The accuracy of the reference centre is dependent upon patient fixation and proper alignment of the instrument (Table 2.2).

Having established a central reference point, rectangular coordinates are given to each data point where a semimeridian intersects a mire. Most commercial systems have 15–38 circular mires and 256–360 equally spaced semimeridians, theoretically providing about 6000–11,000 data points (Fig. 2.7). The actual number of data points available for analysis may be reduced by mire distortion, shadows or the position of the eyelids. The accuracy of the final reconstruction is not dependent

Fig. 2.7 Data points. The data points are located at the intersection of each semimeridian with a ring; for example, a mire composed of 25 rings, each of which is analysed along 256 meridians, will give a total of 6400 potential data points. However, not all data points will be useful as some overlie the eyelids or shadows from the nose or brow and distortion may occur

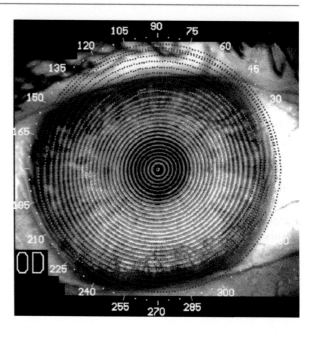

upon the total number of data points, but their density, presuming that each video pixel is not sampled more than once.

Reconstruction Algorithms

Algorithms are the mathematical formulas by which the raw data is converted into topographic information. They reconstruct the three-dimensional shape of the cornea from the two-dimensional image. Their nature varies between different topographic systems, and the details of the formulas vary between commercial models.

The rectangular coordinates locating the data points are converted to polar coordinates on the keratoscope mires to facilitate corneal reconstruction. A reconstruction algorithm [14, 34–39] is then applied to the location of each point on the two-dimensional reflection. This calculates the surface slope at the corneal point from which that reflection originated.

There are two main sources of inaccuracy of reconstruction arising from the algorithm. Firstly, the shape of the normal cornea is complex, and there is no known mathematical formula which exactly describes it. Therefore the algorithm gives only an approximation of the corneal shape and tends to be most accurate centrally where the cornea is more spherical [40]. The second source of inaccuracy is the series of assumptions that have to be made, because each point on the two-dimensional mire image does not represent a unique point in space. For example, for there to be a single solution to the algorithm, it must be assumed that light arising from one meridian on a particular mire falls on the same meridian at the film plane [31, 37, 41] (Table 2.2).

Algorithms vary in the degree of surface smoothing that they incorporate, and some incorporate different levels of smoothing which can be selected by the clinician. The averaging techniques used to achieve smoothing tend to reduce irregularities due to artefacts, but they also underestimate the true irregularities of the surface [25, 28].

Accuracy

Videokeratoscopy measures power of spherical test objects with an accuracy of 0.25D or better within an area equivalent to the central 70% of the corneal surface [17–22] (Table 2.1). This gives a computation accuracy of 0.15D, which is well within any needed clinical tolerance. When measuring radially aspheric surfaces, which are more representative of the normal cornea, accuracy declines very fast in the periphery, dropping to below 3.00D outside a 4 mm radius [23, 28, 40]. This occurs as a result of the spherical bias in the assumptions when calculating the tangential (global) radius of curvature. The peripheral accuracy of videokeratoscopy may be improved by the development of new algorithms [37], shape fitting (e.g. subtracting the corneal shape from a sphere) [42], calculating the instantaneous (local) radius of curvature [40] or matching mathematical equations to the corneal shape.

Accuracy is also reduced for very steep (>46D) or very flat (<38D) corneas [17, 18, 21, 43] and in the presence of marked surface irregularity (Table 2.4).

Checks and Editing

Alignment can be checked in those systems which have the ability to superimpose a semitransparent topography map upon the photokeratoscopy image. If the alignment is not acceptable, the measurement can be repeated. Poor alignment may lead to the erroneous diagnosis of astigmatism, keratoconus or a decentred refractive treatment zone.

Likewise, systems with a side camera can check the position of the corneal apex to confirm that focusing is correct.

Some videokeratoscopes give the clinician the opportunity to edit the acquired image before it is processed. Reflected rings not detected by the computer but visible on the videokeratoscopy image can be completed manually using the mouse. Artefacts, such as the nose, brow and lash shadows, can be eliminated prior to processing. These manoeuvres can improve the cosmetic appearance of a topography map, but they also introduce unreliable data. In most situations it is best to process the image as it was recorded and recognise the cause of artefacts or missing data when interpreting the results. Scheimpflug systems (Chap. 4) are similarly affected by artefacts and missing data [44, 45], but rather than leaving blank areas on the maps, smoothing techniques try to fill in the data, leading to inaccuracies in the representation of irregular corneas.

Display of Results

Once the three-dimensional corneal contour has been reconstructed, the information is displayed in a clinically useful format (Chap. 5).

References

*References Particularly Worth Reading

1. Ambrosio R Jr, Belin MW. Imaging of the cornea: topography vs tomography. J Refract Surg. 2010;26(11):847–9.
2. Dabezies, Halladay. Measurement of corneal curvature: keratometer (ophthalmometer). In: Dabezies OH, Cavanagh HD, Farris RL, et al., editors. Contact lenses: the CLAO guide to basic science and clinical practice. Orlando: Grune and Stratton; 1986.. 17.1–29: Dabezies OH, Halladay JT.
3. Use of the keratometer. In: Bennett AG, editor. Optics of contact lenses. London: ADO publishing; 1974.
4. Gutmark R, Guyton DL. Keratometer and its evolving role in ophthalmology. Surv Ophthalmol. 2010;55(5):481–97.
5. Sunderraj P. Clinical comparison of automated and manual keratometry in pre-operative ocular biometry. Eye. 1992;6:60–2.
6. Cuaycong MJ, Gay CA, Emery J, Haft EA, Koch DD. Comparison of the accuracy of computerized videokeratoscopy and keratometry for use in intraocular lens calculations. J Cataract Refract Surg. 1993;19(Suppl):178–81.
7. Husain SE, Kohnen T, Maturi R, Er H, Koch DD. Computerised videokeratography and keratometry in determining intraocular lens calculations. J Cataract Refract Surg. 1996;22:362–6.
8. Misson GP. Keratometry and postoperative astigmatism. Eye. 1992;6:63–5.
9. *Sanders RD, Gills JP, Martin RG. When keratometric measurements do not accurately reflect corneal topography. J Cataract Refract Surg. 1993;19 Suppl:131–5.
10. Varssano D, Rapuano CJ, Luchs JI. Comparison of keratometric values of healthy and diseased eyes measured by Javal keratometer, EyeSys and PAR. J Cataract Refract Surg. 1997;23:419–22.
11. Rowsey JJ, Reynolds AE, Brown DR. Corneal topography. Corneascope. Arch Ophthalmol. 1981;99:1093–100.
12. Morlet N. Clinical utility of the Barrett keratoscope with astigmatic dial. Ophthalmic Surg. 1994;25:150–3.
13. Maguire LJ, Klyce SD, Sawelson H, McDonald MB, Kaufman HE. Visual distortion after myopic keratomileusis. Computer analysis of keratoscope photographs. Ophthalmic Surg. 1987;18:352–6.
14. Doss JD, Hutson RL, Rowsey JJ, Brown DR. Method for calculation of corneal profile and power distribution. Arch Ophthalmol. 1981;99:1261–5.
15. el Hage SG. A computerized corneal topographer for use in refractive surgery. Refract Corneal Surg. 1989;5:418–24.
16. Keller P, Saarloos PP. Perspectives on corneal topography: a review of videokeratoscopy. Clin Exp Optom. 2009;80(1):18–30.
17. Hannush SB, Crawford SL, Waring GO, Gemmill MC, Lynn MJ, Nizam A. Accuracy and precision of keratometry, photokeratoscopy, and corneal modeling on calibrated steel balls. Arch Ophthalmol. 1989;107:1235–9.
18. Hannush SB, Crawford SL, Waring GO, Gemmill MC, Lynn MJ, Nizam A. Reproducibility of normal corneal power measurements with a keratometer, photokeratoscope, and video imaging system. Arch Ophthalmol. 1990;108:539–44.
19. Wilson SE, Verity SM, Conger DL. Accuracy and precision of the corneal analysis system and the topographical analysis system. Cornea. 1992;11:28–35.
20. Koch DD, Foulks GN, Moran CT, Wakil JS. The corneal EyeSys system: accuracy analysis and reproducibility of first generation prototype. Refract Corneal Surg. 1989;5:424–9.
21. Legeais J-M, Ren Q, Simon G, Parel J-M. Computer-assisted corneal topography: accuracy and reproducibility of the topographic modeling system. Refract Corneal Surg. 1993;9:347–57.

22. Young JA, Talamo JH, Siegel IM. Contour resolution of the EyeSys corneal analysis system. J Cataract Refract Surg. 1995;21:404–6.
23. Douthwaite WA. EyeSys corneal topography measurements applied to calibrated ellipsoidal surfaces. Br J Ophthalmol. 1995;79:797–801.
24. Potvin RJ, Fonn D, Sorbara L. Comparison of polycarbonate and steel test surfaces for video-keratography. J Refract Surg. 1995;11:89–91.
25. Belin MW, Ratliff CD. Evaluating data acquisition and smoothing functions of currently available videokeratoscopes. J Cataract Refract Surg. 1996;22:421–6.
26. Cohen KL, Tripoli NK. Evaluating videokeratoscopes [letter]. J Cataract Refract Surg. 1996;22:871.
27. Belin MW. Evaluating videokeratoscopes [reply]. J Cataract Refract Surg. 1996;22:871–2.
28. *Greivenkamp JE, Mellinger MD, Snyder RW, Schwiegerling JT, Lowman AE, Miller JM. Comparison of three videokeratoscopes in measurement of toric test surfaces. J Refract Surg. 1996;12:229–39.
29. °Zadnik K, Friedman NE, Mutti DO. Repeatability of corneal topography: the "corneal field". J Refract Surg. 1995;11:119–25.
30. Martin R. Cornea and anterior eye assessment with placido-disc keratoscopy, slit scanning evaluation topography and scheimpflug imaging tomography. Indian J Ophthalmol. 2018;66(3):360–6.
31. Wang J, Rice DA, Klyce SD. Analysis of the effects of astigmatism and misalignment on corneal surface reconstruction from photokeratoscopic data. Refract Corneal Surg. 1991;7:129–40.
32. Hubbe RE, Foulks GN. The effect of poor fixation on computer-assisted topographic corneal analysis. Ophthalmology. 1994;101:1745–8.
33. Gao Y, Roberts C. Application of image processing in topographical measurements of the corneal curvature. Proc SPIE. 1994;2132:424–31.
34. Klyce SD. Computer-assisted corneal topography: high resolution graphic presentation and analysis of keratoscopy. Invest Ophthalmol Vis Sci. 1984;25:1426–35.
35. Edmund C, Sjontoft E. The central-peripheral radius of the normal corneal curvature: a photo-keratoscopic study. Acta Ophthalmol. 1985;63:670–7.
36. Maguire LJ, Singer DE, Klyce SD. Graphic presentation of computer analysed keratoscope photographs. Arch Ophthalmol. 1987;105:223–30.
37. Wang J, Rice DA. Klyce SD. A new reconstruction algorithm for improvement of corneal topographical analysis. Refract Corneal Surg. 1989;5:379–87.
38. Tripoli NK, Cohen KL, Holmgren DE, Coggins JM. Assessment of radial aspheres by the arc-step algorithm as implemented by the Keratron keratoscope. Am J Ophthalmol. 1995;120:658–64.
39. *Tripoli NK, Cohen KL, Obla P, Coggins JM, Holmgren DE. Height measurement of astigmatic test surfaces by a keratoscope that uses plane geometry surface reconstruction. Am J Ophthalmol. 1996;121:668–76.
40. °Roberts C. Characterisation of the inherent error in a spherically-biased corneal topography system in mapping a radially aspheric surface. J Refract Corneal Surg. 1994;10:103–11.
41. Arffa RC, Klyce SD, Busin M. Keratometry in epikeratophakia. J Refract Surg. 1989;2:61–4.
42. Stultiens BAT, Jongsma FHM. Frequency modulation as an alternative for local phase in 3D corneal topography. Proc Ophthal Tech. 1994;2126:174–84.
43. Mandell RB. Corneal power correction factor for photorefractive keratectomy. J Cataract Refract Surg. 1994;10:125–8.
44. Wegener A, Laser-Junga H. Photography of the anterior eye segment according to Scheimpflug's principle: options and limitations – a review. Clin Exp Ophthalmol. 2009;37(1):144–54.
45. Oliveira CM, Ribeiro C, Franco S. Corneal imaging with slit-scanning and Scheimpflug imaging techniques. Clin Exp Optom. 2011;94(1):33–42.

Projection-Based Systems

3

A number of corneal topography systems in clinical use today are videokerato-scopes (Chap. 2). These devices are easy to operate and provide useful information, but they rely upon an image being reflected from the corneal surface and therefore have a number of limitations. These are being addressed by the development of topography systems, which utilise the principle of projection. Some projection-based devices have been used mainly in research settings, but it is worth considering them here as they may be the forerunners of techniques developed in the future.

The Principle of Projection

In projection-based methods, an image is formed on the surface of the tear film in the same way as a slide is projected onto a screen (Fig. 3.1).

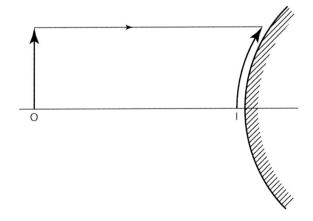

Fig. 3.1 Projected image on the corneal surface. Topography systems using slit photography, rastereography, laser interferometry or moiré interference project an image onto the corneal surface in the same way as a slide is projected onto a screen. Some techniques require the instillation of fluorescein into the tear film (O = object, I = image)

© Springer Nature Switzerland AG 2019
M. Corbett et al., *Corneal Topography*,
https://doi.org/10.1007/978-3-030-10696-6_3

Projection techniques were initially used for sizing industrial machine parts, depth perception in robotics and measurement of body parts in plastic and reconstructive surgery [1].

Application of the technique to the cornea was complicated by two factors. Firstly, the cornea is normally transparent and therefore transmits light, resulting in a low signal. Secondly, light is reflected by the surface of the tear film, resulting in high noise. For the projected image to be visible, it had to be intensified by improving its signal-to-noise ratio.

In the early days of corneal topography, the noise was reduced by applying talcum powder to convert the reflecting tear fluid to an opaque surface. Obviously the application of talcum powder was unacceptable in clinical practice, so attention was turned to increasing the signal. In some systems, this was achieved by adding fluorescein to the tear film to provide image enhancement. However, this is not ideal, because it is not known how the addition of fluorescein alters the normal thickness and distribution of the tear film.

Advantages of Projection-Based Systems

The topography systems dependent upon projection form a less homogeneous group than those using reflection. The general principles apply broadly to most systems (Table 3.1), although there is considerable variation in some of the details.

Measurement of Corneal Height

In contrast to systems using reflection, which measure surface slope, measurements are made in terms of height or elevation above a reference plane. The contours on the corneal map therefore follow lines of equal height, rather than lines of equal slope. Having obtained information in terms of the corneal height, the radius of curvature or corneal power data can then be calculated directly (Chap. 1).

The surface of the normal cornea is very complex, but measurements of corneal height will map its true shape and its normal variations (Chap. 6). It will also help in the understanding of the correlation between corneal topography and visual function.

Table 3.1 Advantages and disadvantages of projection-based topography systems compared to reflection-based systems (e.g. videokeratoscopes)

Advantages	Disadvantages
Corneal height measurements	Prototype less easy to use
Irregular surfaces measured	Image acquisition longer in some
Non-reflective surfaces measured	Image analysis longer in some
Entire corneal area measured	Less clinical experience to date
High resolution and accuracy	No standardised presentation formats
Uniform accuracy across cornea	Fluorescein instillation in some
Lack of spherical bias	

Knowledge of the true corneal shape is helpful in the fitting of therapeutic contact lenses, when the posterior lens surface has to encompass all protuberances on the anterior corneal surface (Chap. 7). There may also be a role in the monitoring of corneal disease, such as the size or depth of a corneal ulcer or gutter (Chaps. 8, 9 and 10).

Measurements of corneal height are also useful in planning refractive surgery, such as photorefractive keratectomy or LASIK. The refractive outcome of these procedures is highly dependent upon the precise depth of tissue removed by the ablation process and the amount of newly synthesised tissue laid down on this surface during wound healing (Chap. 14).

Corneal height measured immediately postoperative provides information about the spatial uniformity of the excimer laser beam and the profile of the ablation [2, 3]. Subtraction of the immediate postoperative topography from subsequent maps quantifies new tissue production at intervals during the healing process [4]. Measures such as these are important in characterising the wound healing response and objectively comparing the results of different ablation profiles or postoperative drug treatments.

In some patients, it is possible to use this information to treat irregular corneal astigmatism using the excimer laser. The true corneal shape map can be used in two ways. Most commonly it is coupled directly to a small-diameter "flying spot" laser in which it controls the location of the beam. Less frequently these days, the height information can be used to lathe an individualised erodible mask whose shape is complementary to that of the cornea. As the mask is ablated, more corneal tissue is removed from the high areas where the mask was thinnest than the low areas where the mask was thickest. This would create a more spherical or normally shaped surface. In theory, the technique would be particularly useful in the retreatment of decentred ablation zones and conditions such as keratoconus. However, such cases require symmetry of the wound healing processes if these shape changes are to be maintained, and other factors such as the thickness of the cornea and risk of an abnormal healing response would need to be considered prior to deciding to proceed with treatment.

Irregular and Non-reflective Surfaces

Projection-based systems have wider applications than videokeratoscopy in corneal disease, because they can make measurements from irregular or non-reflective surfaces. They are able to provide information about the true morphology of a number of corneal pathologies and may give some insight into their nature and progression.

One important benefit arising from the ability of these systems to make measurements from non-reflective surfaces is that information can be obtained about the corneal surface immediately after laser refractive surgery. This is necessary in any investigation of ablation profiles or postoperative wound healing.

It could also provide a potential means of measuring the shape of the corneal surface during the ablation procedure itself and during other surgical procedures [3]. This may be useful in the tailoring of treatments to individual patients.

Entire Corneal Coverage

Projection-based systems are able to make measurements from the whole cornea, including the very centre and the limbus. The accuracy of the reconstruction is maintained out to the periphery, and therefore detailed information about this area can be provided.

The topography of the very centre of the cornea is important due to its role in vision. It is also important to be able to study the shape of the corneal periphery to monitor wound construction (e.g. in new techniques such as femtosecond laser) as well as peripheral corneal pathology such as peripheral ulcerative keratitis, corneal melt and gutters, which tend to occur preferentially in the perilimbal area.

High Resolution and Accuracy

Using projection-based methods, it is possible to achieve a resolution higher than with videokeratoscopes. For some devices, the resolution is in the order of 2–5 μm.

The reconstruction of the corneal shape from projection-derived data is of uniform accuracy across the whole cornea. It lacks spherical bias as the analysis is not performed with relation to the visual axis or the centre of the cornea. Therefore the alignment of the cornea for capture of the image is less important than for videokeratoscopes.

Focusing is also less important as these systems tend to use parallel light. In addition, the surface is reconstructed from the position of the points relative to each other and the mathematical reference plane, rather than at an absolute position in space. Therefore these systems are potentially less prone to operator error.

Disadvantages of Projection-Based Systems

Influence of Tear Fluid

Both reflection- and projection-based topography systems image the air-tear fluid interface rather than the surface of the corneal epithelium. As topography systems become more accurate, it is necessary to consider how the tear fluid influences measurements.

Both types of system rely upon the assumption that the tear fluid is a thin layer of uniform thickness covering the entire surface from which measurements are made. Early estimates of tear film thickness were about 7 μm [5], which would have negligible effect on the corneal curvature or power and is well below the sensitivity of currently available videokeratoscopes, which have and accuracy of 0.25D in the central region.

However, more recent studies have found the tear film to be thicker, with some reports claiming 40 μm [6], and the uniformity is unknown. In this situation the tear film could potentially affect topography, particularly as measurement techniques become more sensitive. This degree of sensitivity is now achievable, as some systems have an axial resolution of at least 5 μm and can reconstruct the inferior tear meniscus. The viscosity of the tear fluid may serve to integrate out microundulations in the corneal surface by being thicker over depressions and thinner over protuberances. However, this is unlikely to be of clinical importance, as it is the air-tear fluid interface which is the major refractive surface of the eye.

Some devices require the instillation of fluorescein into the tear fluid to enhance the signal-to-noise ratio during image acquisition. The effects of this on corneal topography are unknown but are unlikely to be significant following the small quantities used.

Lack of Standardised Presentation Formats

With the development of new topography systems and methods of data analysis, there is an increasing number of ways in which topographic information is presented [7] (Chap. 5). Each presentation format may have its individual merits, but there could be considerable benefits in developing a standard format [8] which could be chosen as a presentation option in all systems. At this time of rapid expansion in the field of corneal topography, we should perhaps be considering whether this is the most useful format. We should also consider whether more than one standardised format will ultimately be required to present the wealth of information which can now be obtained about corneal topography. Given the problems which occurred in developing standards in electrophysiology and perimetry, the need for an internationally agreed system may be rapidly approaching.

Slit Photography

When observing the cornea on the slit lamp using a narrow beam, the shape of the anterior and posterior corneal surfaces in one meridian can be seen due to the curved appearance of the beam (Fig. 3.2). If a slit beam scans across the cornea, 40 independent images can be recorded from a known angle by a calibrated video camera. Each slit contains up to 240 data points, giving a total of over 9000 data points on each surface, each with a resolution of 2 μm [9].

The reconstruction algorithms can generate a map of the entire anterior and posterior surfaces. In addition, subtraction of these two maps can provide a map of corneal thickness. This is particularly useful in corneal diseases, such as keratoconus and peripheral gutters, and in the planning of incisional refractive surgery and laser in situ keratomileusis (LASIK).

Limitations of this technology include the relatively long time (0.8 seconds) required to individually image 40 slits and the resultant possibility of introducing artefacts due to eye movement. A number of studies have illustrated this device is potentially inaccurate at locating the posterior corneal surface and hence tends to underestimate corneal thickness after refractive surgery [10–18].

Fig. 3.2 Corneal slit. When a narrow slit of light shines on the cornea, the anterior and posterior surfaces can be seen in the beam. When viewed from a known angle, the shape of these two surfaces in that plane can be determined and the corneal thickness calculated. The information from multiple parallel slits can be combined to reconstruct the entire cornea

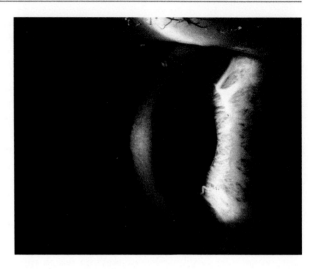

In the future, if the magnification and resolution of the images can be improved, there is the potential for this device to measure not only total corneal thickness but also corneal epithelial thickness. This would be valuable in research in refractive surgery and clinically when deciding how to retreat patients who regress after treatment. A technique with a similar aim is the measurement of corneal and epithelial thickness using high-frequency ultrasonography [19, 20].

Rasterstereography

In rasterstereography (or rasterphotogrammetry), a grid is projected onto the tear film surface and imaged from a known angle [21–25]. The topographic elevation is calculated from the displacement of components within the grid image when projected onto the corneal surface, compared to their known position when projected onto a flat surface (Fig. 3.3).

The number of data points used by this method was initially limited by the number of grid intersections. However, a far greater number of data points can be obtained if the lines of the grid have a sine wave function, and the greyscale value of each pixel is measured to detect local changes in grating intensity [26, 27].

Moiré Interference

Moiré interference occurs when two sets of parallel lines are superimposed at different orientations, as seen, for example, when two net curtains overlap [28, 29]. When parallel gratings (Fig. 3.4a) are projected obliquely onto a cornea, the image on the corneal surface is a series of parallel lines, curved in a similar manner to that seen when using a slit lamp beam (Fig. 3.4b). Gratings projected from

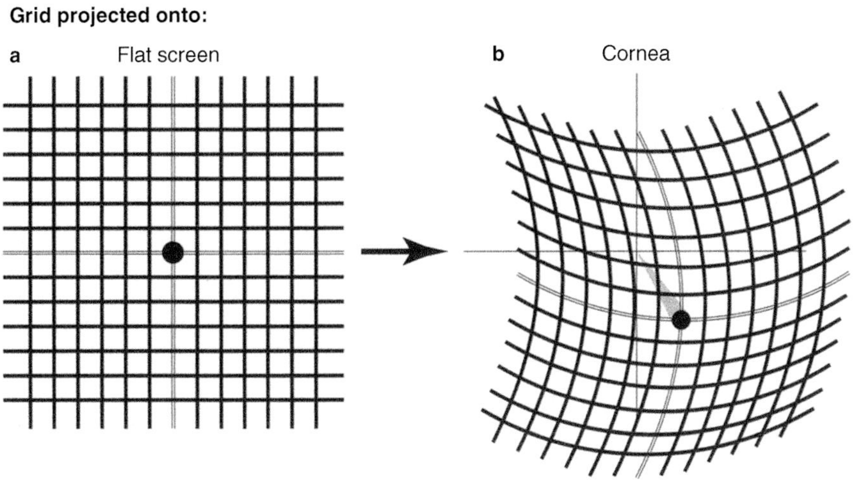

Grid projected onto:

a   Flat screen   b   Cornea

Fig. 3.3 Rastereography. Diagrammatic representation of the measurement of corneal height by rastereography (rasterphotogrammetry). A grid is projected onto the tear film surface from a known angle. The topographic elevation is calculated from the displacement of components within the grid image when projected onto the corneal surface (**b**), compared to their known position when projected onto a flat surface (**a**)

the nasal and temporal sides produced images curved in opposite directions. Addition of these two images results in moiré interference which generates ring-shaped interference fringes visible on the corneal surface (Figs. 3.4c and 3.5). These fringes follow contour lines representing points of equal height (Fig. 3.4d) and can be viewed directly without recourse to mathematical assumptions or computations [30, 31].

The width of the moiré fringes is partially determined by the spatial frequency of the gratings. Their orientation is dependent upon the relative orientations of the two grating images and therefore the shape of the surface on which they are formed. As with rasterstereography, if the gratings have a sine wave function [26, 27], a huge number of data points can be generated (e.g. more than 200,000), with a very high resolution in the z-axis (<5 μm).

Laser Interferometry

Interferometry records the interference pattern generated on the corneal surface by the interference of two coherent wave fronts [31–35]. The two wave fronts may be generated by light from separate illuminating and reference lasers, or the light from an illuminating laser may be directed through two distinct optical pathways by the use of a beam splitter. The corneal elevation is calculated from analysis of the interference pattern (Fig. 3.6). The density of data points generated is dependent upon the wavelength of the light.

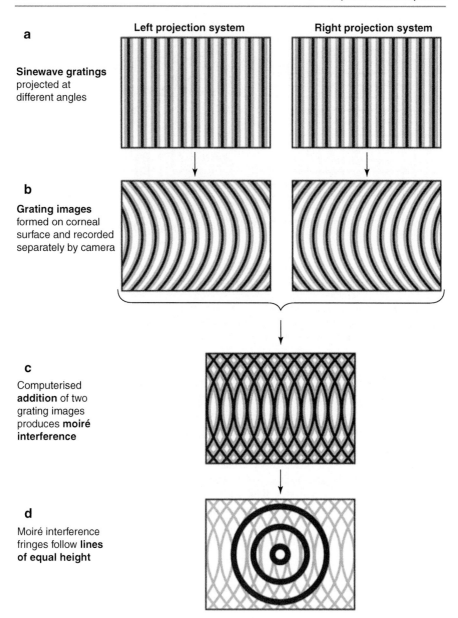

Fig. 3.4 Moiré interference. Diagrammatic representation of the generation of moiré interference fringes. Two parallel sine wave gratings (**a**) are projected at equal and opposite angles to the visual axis. The light approaches the cornea obliquely, and therefore the lines of the grating images formed on the corneal surface appear curved (**b**). Addition of the two images results in moiré interference (**c**), in which the ring-shaped interference fringes follow contour lines representing points of equal height (**d**)

Fig. 3.5 Moiré interference fringes. Circular moiré interference patterns on the corneal surface are formed by the computerised addition of two sine wave grating images. The fringes follow lines of equal height, but as there are so few rings generated, detailed shape information is provided by the computer analysis of the sine wave grating on the two individual images

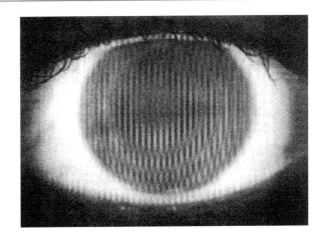

Fig. 3.6 Laser interferometry. Holographic interferogram of an eyebank cornea with four deep radial incisions. (Courtesy of Dr Smolek, Louisiana State University, Lions Eye Centre. Adapted from *Journal of Cataract and Refractive Surgery* 1994;20:282)

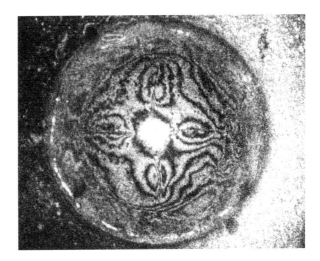

References

References Particularly Worth Reading

1. Warnicki JW, Rehkopf PG, Arrra RC, Stuart JC. Corneal topography using a projected grid. In: Schanzlin DJ, Robin JB, editors. Corneal topography. Measuring and modifying the cornea. New York: Springer; 1992. p. 25–32.
2. Liang F-Q, Geasey SD, del Cerro Maquavella JV. A new procedure for evaluating smoothness of corneal surface following 193nm excimer laser ablation. Refract Corneal Surg. 1992;8:459–65.
3. Ediger MN, Pettit GH, Weiblinger RP. Noninvasive monitoring of excimer laser ablation by time-resolved reflectometry. Refract Corneal Surg. 1993;9:268–75.

4. Corbett MC, Verma S, Prydal JI, Pande M, Oliver KM, Patel S, Marshall J. The contribution of the corneal epithelium to the refractive changes occurring after excimer laser photorefractive keratectomy. Invest Ophthalmol Vis Sci. 1995;36:S2.
5. Mishima S. Some physiological aspects of the precorneal tearfilm. Arch Ophthalmol. 1965;73:233.
6. Prydal JI, Campbell FW. Study of precorneal tear film thickness and structure by interferometry and confocal microscopy. Invest Ophthalmol Vis Sci. 1992;33:1996–2005.
7. Naufal SC, Hess JS, Friedlander MH, Granet NS. Rasterstereography-based classification of normal corneas. J Cataract Refract Surg. 1997;23:222–30.
8. Wilson SE, Klyce SD, Husseini ZM. Standardized color-coded maps for corneal topography. Ophthalmology. 1993;100:1723–7.
9. *Auffarth GU, Tetz MR, Biazid Y, Völcker HE. Measuring anterior chamber depth with the Orbscan topography system. J Cataract Refract Surg. 1997;23(9):1351–5.
10. Cairns G, Ormonde SE, Gray T, et al. Assessing the accuracy of the Orbscan II post LASIK: apparent keratectasia is paradoxically associated with anterior chamber depth reduction in successful procedures. Clin Exp Ophthalmol. 2005;33:147–52.
11. Cairns G, McGhee CN. Orbscan computerised topography: attributes, applications and limitations. J Cataract Refract Surg. 2005;31:205–20.
12. Hashemi H, Mehravaran S. Corneal changes after laser refractive surgery for myopia: comparison of Orbscan II and Pentacam findings. J Cataract Refract Surg. 2007;33:841–7.
13. Prisant O, Calderon N, Chastang P, et al. Reliability of pachymetric measurements using Orbscan after excimer refractive surgery. Ophthalmology. 2003;110:511–5.
14. Kamiya K, Oshika T, Amano S, et al. Influence of excimer laser PRK on the posterior corneal surface. J Cataract Refract Surg. 2000;26:867–71.
15. Naroo SA, Charman WN. Changes in posterior corneal curvature after PRK. J Cataract Refract Surg. 2000;26:872–8.
16. Seitz B, Torres F, Langenbucher A, et al. Posterior corneal curvature changes after myopic LASIK. Ophthalmology. 2001;108:666–72.
17. Wang Z, Chen J, Yang B. Posterior corneal surface topography changes after LASIK are related to residual corneal bed thickness. Ophthalmology. 1999;106:406–9.
18. Baek T, Lee K, Kagaya F, et al. Factors affecting the forward shift of posterior corneal surface after LASIK. Ophthalmology. 2001;108:317–20.
19. Reinstein DZ, Silverman RH, Coleman J. High-frequency ultrasound measurement of the thickness of the corneal epithelium. Refract Corneal Surg. 1993;9:385–7.
20. Reinstein DZ, Archer TJ, Gobbe M, Silverman RH, Coleman DJ. Epithelial thickness in the normal cornea: three-dimensional display with Artemis very high-frequency digital ultrasound. J Refract Surg. 2008;24(6):571–81.
21. Warnicki JW, Rehkopf PG, Curtin DY, Burns SA, Arffa RC, Stuart JC. Corneal topography using computer analyzed rasterstereographic images. Appl Opt. 1988;27:1135–40.
22. *Arffa RC, Warnicki JW, Rehkopf PG. Corneal topography using rastereography. Refract Corneal Surg. 1989;5:414–7.
23. *Belin MW, Litoff FK, Strods SJ, Winn SS, Smith RS. The PAR technology corneal topography system. Refract Corneal Surg. 1992;8:88–96.
24. Belin MW. Intraoperative raster photogrammetry – the PAR Corneal Topography System. J Cataract Refract Surg. 1993;19(Suppl):188–92.
25. Belin MW, Zloty P. Accuracy of the PAR corneal topography system with spatial misalignment. CLAO J. 1993;19:64–8.
26. Stultiens BAT, Jongsma FHM. Frequency modulation as an alternative for local phase in 3D corneal topography. Proc Ophthal Tech. 1994;2126:174–84.
27. Takeda M, Ina H, Kobayashi S. Fourier-transform method of fringe-pattern analysis for computer-based topography and interferometry. J Opt Soc Am. 1982;72:156–60.
28. Corbett MC, O'Brart DPS, Stultiens BAT, Jongsma FHM, Marshall J. Corneal topography using a new moiré image-based system. Eur J Implant Ref Surg. 1995;7:353–70.

29. *Jongsma FHM, Laan FC, Stultiens BATh. A moiré based corneal topographer suitable for discrete Fourier analysis. Proc Ophthal Tech. 1994;2126:185–92.
30. Kawara T. Corneal topography using moire contour fringes. Appl Opt. 1979;18:3675–8.
31. Varner JR. Holographic and moiré surface contouring. In: Erf R, editor. Holographic non-destructive testing. New York: Academic Press; 1974. p. 105–47.
32. Skolnick AA. New holographic process provides noninvasive, 3-D anatomic views. JAMA. 1994;271:5–8.
33. *Smolek MK. Holographic interferometry of intact and radially incised human eye-bank corneas. J Cataract Refract Surg. 1994;20:277–86.
34. Baker PC. Holographic contour analysis of the cornea. In: Masters BR, editor. Non-invasive diagnostic techniques in ophthalmology. New York: Springer-Verlag; 1990. p. 82–97.
35. Kasprzak H, Kowalik W, Jaronski J. Inferometric measurements of fine corneal curvature. SPIE. 1994;2329:32–9.

Scheimpflug Camera-Based Systems

4

Introduction

Imaging of the cornea and anterior segment has advanced significantly in recent years allowing a greater understanding of the structure and refractive function of the front of the eye. An important class of devices is the Scheimpflug camera-based systems, which permit detailed mapping of the anterior and posterior corneal surface, the measurement of corneal pachymetry and a number of other anterior chamber parameters. Applications include the diagnosis of anterior segment pathology with monitoring of disease progression, pre- and post-refractive surgery assessment and research.

The Scheimpflug Principle

The Scheimpflug principle is a geometric rule that enables the photographer to capture sharp, focused images of objects that are not parallel to the camera and lens. It enables an enhanced depth of focus without distorting the image and is commonly used in photography. Originally described by Jules Carpentier in 1901, the principle is named after Austrian army Captain Theodor Scheimpflug, who used it to devise a systematic method and apparatus for correcting perspective distortion in aerial photographs [1]. However, it was not until the 1970s that a group of researchers led by Professor Otto Hockwin developed a Scheimpflug slit-imaging device for ophthalmological use.

The principle describes the orientation of the plane of focus of an optical system when the object plane, lens plane and the image plane are not parallel but intersect at a common point in space. Ideally the lens and the image plane are parallel: a linear object will form a plane of focus parallel to the lens plane and thus can be completely in focus on the image plane (Fig. 4.1a). When the object is not parallel to the image plane, it is not possible to focus the entire image on a plane parallel to image plane (Fig. 4.1b), which may lead to image blur and distortion. Using the

© Springer Nature Switzerland AG 2019
M. Corbett et al., *Corneal Topography*,
https://doi.org/10.1007/978-3-030-10696-6_4

Fig. 4.1 Illustration of the Scheimpflug principle, using the examples of (**a**) parallel object, lens and image; (**b**) object, lens and image planes not parallel; and (**c**) the Scheimpflug intersection. (Scheimpflug T. 1904; Adapted from EyeWiki.aao.org; Zeimer website: http://www.ziemergroup.com/products/galilei/product-profile/theory/scheimpflug.html)

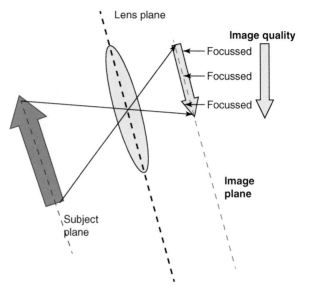

a

Subject plane, lens plane and image plane are parallel, thus creating a sharp focus overall

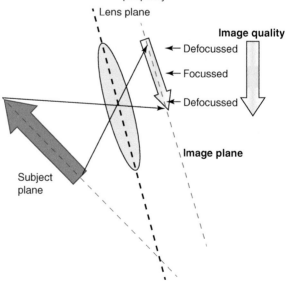

b

Subject plane is not parallel to image plane, poor focus at periphery

Fig. 4.1 (continued)   c

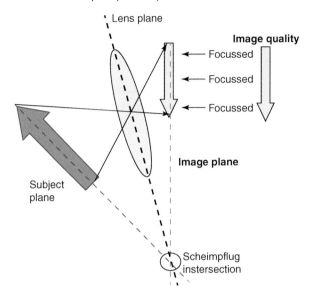

Subject plane is still not parallel to image plane, however image plane is manipulated according to Scheimpflug principle: sharp focus overall

Scheimpflug principle, an oblique tangent can be drawn from the image, object and lens planes, and their point of convergence is called the Scheimpflug intersection (Fig. 4.1c). Careful movement of the image and lens planes can lead to a focused and sharp image on the entire non-parallel object. This has obvious advantages and uses for imaging a curved object such as the cornea.

Scheimpflug-Based Systems

Single Scheimpflug Imaging

One of the first commercially available systems to incorporate this technology was the Pentacam™ (Oculus GmbH). It obtains images of the anterior segment using a rotating Scheimpflug digital CCD camera and a light source of UV-free blue LEDs with a wavelength of 475 nm. It rotates around a central axis and captures 50 meridional pictures, each passing through a common point at the centre of the cornea. The Pentacam software extracts 500 elevation points from each image, obtaining 25,000 true elevation points from each corneal surface. Measurements take less than 2 s, and the system is able to realign the central thinnest point of each section before it reconstructs the corneal image, which minimises any movement-related artefact. In addition, it is possible to examine each individual meridional image to look for a blinking eyelid or patient misalignment that might degrade the image.

Scheimpflug photography provides images of the anterior segment with minimal distortion from the camera optics, cornea and lens. Correction of any image distortion is important when assessing corneal biometry, refractive surgery, anterior chamber biometry and for control of intraocular lens position stability. It is less significant for measurement of the light-scattering profile and aberrations in the cornea and lens.

Most of the biometrical measurements obtained (corneal curvature, change of lens curvature with accommodation, depth of anterior chamber, anterior chamber angle) have to be optimised using algorithms [2, 3]. The Pentacam is a tomographer, and its software incorporates a ray-tracing algorithm to construct and calculate a mathematical three-dimensional image of the entire anterior segment. It can also evaluate both the anterior and posterior surfaces to create an accurate pachymetric map for the entire cornea.

Image analysis is achieved via linear densitometry and correlates the density to a certain layer of the cornea and lens. This allows discrimination of the different layers by density quantification with analysis influenced by a variety of factors such as pupil size and light intensity. Variation in these parameters will affect the accuracy of the data such that a degree of standardisation is necessary. It has enabled the generation of normative databases for topographic parameters useful in corneal and refractive surgery [4].

Dual Scheimpflug Imaging

Dual Scheimpflug camera-based systems utilise two Scheimpflug cameras orientated at 90° to each other that rotate around a common central axis containing the slit beam light source (see Fig. 4.2). The principal advantage of this design is that it allows corresponding corneal data from each channel to be compared and averaged to compensate for unintentional misalignment and eye movement. It is not influenced by angular surfaces, which allows it to calculate accurate pachymetry even when the degree of decentration from the corneal apex is unknown. It is able to place each averaged thickness and posterior height value to its proper location in the cornea, whereas single Scheimpflug systems have to make estimations on the variable surface inclination before calculating correct thicknesses or posterior heights. This is illustrated by a study, which showed single-camera devices are more precise for curvature, astigmatism and corneal wavefront error measurements and the dual-camera device for pachymetry measurements [5].

The two Scheimpflug channels are positioned opposite each other and aligned symmetrically to the rotational axis containing the slit beam. When the machine is centred on the corneal apex, the apparent thicknesses of both camera views are identical. If the slit beam is positioned off-centre, the optics will be inclined to the corneal surface resulting in two apparent slit images, which are deviated, from each

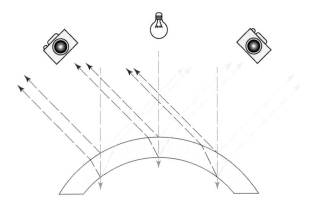

Fig. 4.2 Illustration of the dual Scheimpflug principle. Averaging of the thicknesses in the two corresponding Scheimpflug views (green and blue lines) reduces the decentration error by a factor of 10, without the need for correcting the misalignment. This error can range from 30 μm at 1 mm to 10 μm at 0.3 mm decentration, which is well within the range of normal eye movements during target fixation. (Adapted from Galilei Dual Scheimpflug Analyzer. Zeimer Ophthalmology 2008)

other. The reciprocal dual-camera views allow averaging of these corresponding values to correct any error from the misalignment. Given the natural movement of human eyes in vivo, this system facilitates more accurate mapping of the cornea and anterior segment.

Integration of Placido Topography

Two corneal curves with a difference of 0.25 dioptres have the same elevation at the centre but will gradually separate towards the periphery. Within the central 1 mm diameter region, the maximum difference in elevation is 0.1 μm, but at 3 mm diameter region, this has increased to 0.9 μm. In order to distinguish between these two curves using a slit beam, the pixel resolution must be extremely high [6, 7]. The problem is magnified using a Scheimpflug image as the corneal curvature is only a small proportion of the anterior segment image. This is overcome by integrating infrared Placido topography with dual Scheimpflug imaging. Several devices incorporate both technologies with the aim of improving accuracy in central anterior corneal curvature measurements.

Advantages of Scheimpflug-Based Systems

Scheimpflug-based topography has significantly improved imaging in ophthalmology, enabling clinicians to obtain optical sections of the entire anterior segment of the eye, from the anterior surface of the cornea to the posterior surface of the lens. Using a wide depth of focus, assessment of anterior and posterior corneal topography, anterior and posterior topography of the lens as well as anterior chamber depth is achieved.

The rotation of the imaging process around the central cornea has several advantages over scanning slit systems using parallel images. These include:

(a) Precise measurement of the central cornea
(b) Ability to correct for small eye movements
(c) Easy fixation for patient
(d) Short examination time

Measurements take around 2 s, and minute eye movements are captured and corrected simultaneously. Using 3D image stitching, it is possible to measure 25,000 true elevation points precisely and reproducibly. Using computer algorithms and mathematical models, it can calculate:

(a) Anterior and posterior corneal elevation maps
(b) Keratometry (K) readings
(c) Corneal pachymetry from limbus to limbus
(d) 3D chamber analysing (anterior chamber depth map, chamber angle, chamber volume)
(e) Lens density (quantification of the light transmittance of the crystalline lens and IOL)
(f) Tomography
(g) Improved IOL calculation for post LASIK, photo refractive keratotomy and radial keratotomy patients

The rotating Scheimpflug device does not appear to suffer from the same limitations as the scanning slit device (see Chap. 3) with regard to post-refractive measurements [8–14].

Disadvantages of Scheimpflug-Based Systems

Calculation of corneal power from elevation measurements has several limitations.

The use of elevation data to represent the corneal elevation data in comparison to a reference surface results in points being labelled as higher or lower than the reference plane. The points higher are depicted on colour-coded maps as red, whilst those that drop below the reference surface are shown in blue. This can lead to confusions when comparing with a Placido-based corneal power map, because the areas with a steeper curvature or higher dioptric power are shown in red, whilst flatter curvatures and lesser powers are shown in blue.

A comparison of accuracy of the different Scheimpflug machines is not possible as there is no gold standard. In addition, each machine uses different algorithms and systems to extrapolate and calculate data. Galilei has changed the optical reference plane for the definition of corneal power to the anterior corneal surface decreasing its value by about 3% with respect to previous versions. Pentacam calculates total corneal refractive power in relation to the posterior corneal surface. So, even if names and definitions on the software are similar, they employ different parameters, and care must be taken in their use.

In addition, Scheimpflug imaging may be biased by imperfections in cornea clarity and epithelial irregularities, resulting in false positive changes to the posterior corneal surface and pachymetry.

Hence, the ultimate solution may be to use both a Placido-based image analysis for corneal power requirements and to interpret these in light of data above corneal elevation from devices like the Pentacam – for both the anterior and posterior corneal surfaces.

Other Applications

Corvis® ST

The Corvis® ST (Oculus) records the deformation of the cornea to a defined air pulse using a high-speed Scheimpflug camera that captures over 4300 images per second. This allows a precise measurement of IOP and corneal thickness based on the Scheimpflug images taken [15]. One hundred and forty images are taken within 31 ms after onset of the air pulse and converted into a video. The recorded deformation of the cornea allows its biomechanical properties to be studied in more detail and has significant implications for the management of corneal disease and laser refractive surgery [16].

Whilst measurements are highly reproducible, some studies have shown significant differences in measurement parameters between other types of device [17], whilst others have shown no statistically significant difference in compared biometric parameters between a Scheimpflug device (Pentacam), a swept-source optical biometer (IOL Master 700) and a standard optical biometer (IOL Master 500) [18].

References

1. Scheimpflug T. Improved method and apparatus for the systematic alteration or distortion of plane pictures and images by means of lenses and mirrors for photography and for other purposes. GB Patent No. 1196. Filed 16 January 1904, and issued 12 May 1904.
2. Dubbellman M, Van Der Heijde RGL. The shape of the aging human lens: curvature, equivalent refractive index and the lens paradoxon. Vis Res. 2001;41:1867–88.
3. Dubbellman M, Weeber HA, Van Der Heijde RGL, Volker-Dieben HJ. Radius and asphericity of the posterior corneal surface determined by corrected Scheimpflug photography. Acta Ophthalmol Scand. 2002;80:379–83.
4. Gilani F, Cortese M, Ambrósio RR Jr, et al. Comprehensive anterior segment normal values generated by rotating Scheimpflug tomography. J Cataract Refract Surg. 2013;39(11):1707–12.
5. Aramberri J, Araiz L. Garcia A. et al. Dual versus single Scheimpflug camera for anterior segment analysis: precision and agreement. J Cataract Refract Surg 2012;38(11):1934–1949.
6. Mandell RB, St. Helen R. Stability of the corneal contour. Am J Optom. 1968;45(12):797–806.
7. Roberts C. . The resolution necessary for surface height measurements of the cornea. Optical Society of America Annual Meeting, October 2–7 1994.

8. Ciolino JB, Belin MW. Changes in the posterior cornea after LASIK and PRK. J Caract Refract Surg. 2006;32:1426–31.

9. Buehl W, Sojanac D, Sacu S, et al. Comparison of three methods of measuring corneal thickness and anterior chamber depth. Am J Ophthalmol. 2006;141:7–12.

10. Lackner B, Schmidinger C, Pieh S, et al. Repeatability and reproducibility of central corneal thickness measurement with Pentacam, Orbscan and ultrasound. Optom Vis Sci. 2005;82:892–9.

11. Lackner B, Schmidinger C, Skorpic C. Validity and repeatability of anterior chamber depth measurements with Pentacam and Orbscan. Optom Vis Sci. 2005;82:858–61.

12. O'Donnell C, Maldonado-Codina C. Agreement and repeatability of central thickness measurement in normal corneas using ultrasound pachymetry and the Oculus Pentacam. Cornea. 2005;24:920–4.

13. Ucakhan OO, Ozkan M, Kanpolat A. Corneal thickness measurements in normal and keratoconic eyes: Pentacam comprehensive eye scanner versus non-contact specular microscopy and ultrasound pachymetry. J Cataract Refract Surg. 2006;32:970–7.

14. Ciolino JB, Khachikian SS, Cortese MJ, Belin MW. Long-term stability of the posterior cornea after LASIK. J Cataract Refract Surg. 2007;33:1366–70.

15. Salvetat ML, Zeppieri M, Tosoni C, et al. Corneal deformation parameters provided by the Corvis-ST Pachy-tonometer in healthy subjects and glaucoma patients. J Glaucoma. 2015;24(8):568–74.

16. Roberts CJ. Importance of accurately assessing biomechanics of the cornea. Curr Opin Ophthalmol. 2016;27(4):285–91.

17. Sel S, Stange J, Kaiser D, et al. Repeatability and agreement of Scheimpflug-based and swept-source optical biometry measurements. Cont Lens Anterior Eye. 2017;40(5):318–22.

18. Shajari M, Cremonese C, Petermann K, et al. Comparison of axial length, corneal curvature, and anterior chamber depth measurements of 2 recently introduced devices to a known biometer. Am J Ophthalmol. 2017;178:58–64.

Presentation of Topographic Information

5

The aim of corneal topography is to obtain detailed, accurate data about the corneal contour and display it in a clinically useful format [1, 2]. The raw image captured by topography systems often only reveals to the observer relatively gross abnormalities of corneal structure. For example, alterations in the shape or spacing of videokeratoscopy mires are only apparent for astigmatism greater than 3.00D. Computer analysis of the raw image quantifies the corneal contour and displays the data in formats which are much more sensitive to small abnormalities of the surface [3, 4].

All topography systems have many formats in which its data can be displayed. The key to maximising the information obtained from a topography examination is to select the most appropriate display format. Each format has certain benefits, limitations and applications, which are described below.

When presented with a topography display (Fig. 5.1), it should be studied in structured fashion in order to obtain the maximum information from it and avoid mistakes in interpretation (Table 5.1). The same system can be applied to any form of topographic display, produced by any device. If the display is being studied in conjunction with a patient, the name, date, eye and other detail should first be confirmed from the patient and examination information sections. The scale should then be studied to determine the type of measurement and the step interval. Only then should the map itself be studied.

Interpretation of the map is performed largely on the application of a few basic principles *(see below)* and pattern recognition *(see later chapters)*. This can be aided by studying any statistical information provided. Comparison can be made with previous topography examinations of the same eye. It is also sometimes useful to compare the topography of the other eye, as pairs of normal corneas are often mirror images of each other. However, in both these situations, care should be taken to express all the sets of data with the same scales, so like can be compared with like.

© Springer Nature Switzerland AG 2019
M. Corbett et al., *Corneal Topography*,
https://doi.org/10.1007/978-3-030-10696-6_5

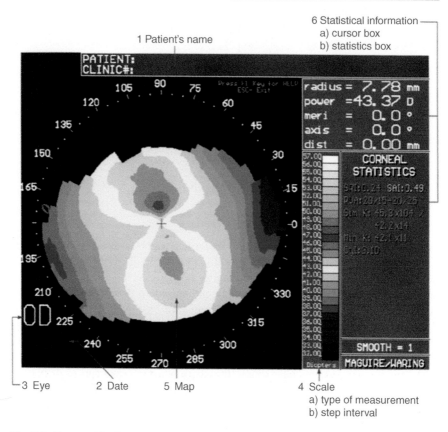

Fig. 5.1 Topographic display. A typical topographic display composed of several parts, which should be studied systematically in the order shown

Table 5.1 System for studying topographic displays. When presented with a topographic display, it must be studied systematically to maximise the information obtained and avoid mistakes in interpretation	System for studying topography displays
	Check name, date, eye
	Scale:
	Type of measurement (e.g. height, curvature, power)
	Step interval
	Map
	Statistical information, (e.g. cursor box, indices)
	Compare previous maps of the same eye (check that the scale is the same)
	Compare with topography of the other eye (check that the scale is the same)

Measurements

The types of measurements which can be made by topography systems have been described in Chap. 1.

Raw Image

The study of the raw image captured by the camera in the topography device can provide extra clinical information which is of use in the interpretation of the map (Fig. 5.2). For example, the demonstration of focal irregularities, which correspond to surface pathology or tear film abnormalities.

Height

Height data is immediately available from systems using the principle of projection. It is very useful in numeric or cross-sectional format (Fig. 5.3a), because it can precisely quantify the elevation of a proud nebula or the depth of an excimer laser ablation or ulcer [5]. A three-dimensional height map gives a good concept of the overall shape of the cornea, but more subtle details are not obvious [6] (Fig. 5.3c).

A more sensitive way of presenting height data is to plot the difference in height from a sphere of known size [1, 2, 7] or from an idealised corneal shape. This is

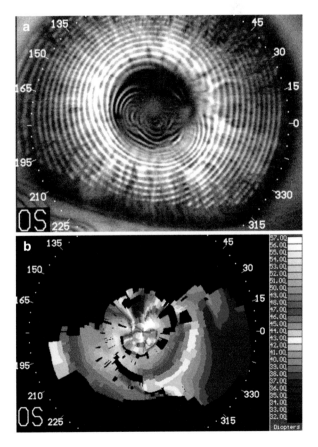

Fig. 5.2 Videokeratograph. Severe keratoconus in which there are two proud nebulae superior to the apex of the cone. The raw image (**a**) shows the irregularity which prevents reliable reconstruction of the topography on the colour map (**b**). Maps of the same eye using different techniques are shown in Figs. 5.3 and 5.5

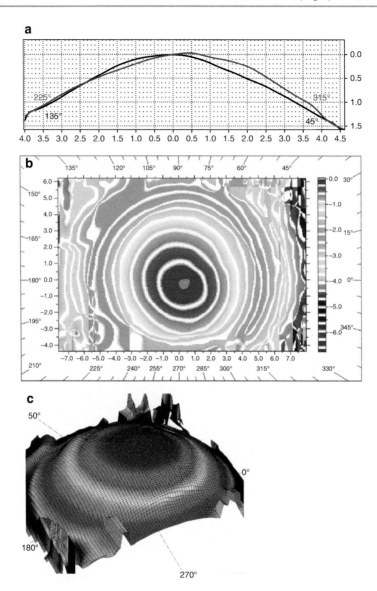

Fig. 5.3 Corneal height. The same left eye with keratoconus and an inferotemporal cone. The corneal height has been measured by a projection-based system using moiré interference and Fourier analysis. (**a**) A cross section is a one-dimensional representation of the corneal height (mm). The 45° meridian (black) has a relatively normal, symmetrical shape. The 135° meridian (red) is flattened superonasally and protrudes more than normal in the inferotemporal quadrant. The apex of the cone in that meridian is 0.45 mm from the corneal centre (visual axis). (**b**) The two-dimensional representation of corneal height demonstrated only relatively gross abnormalities. The contours appear closest together where the cornea is steepest inferotemporally. The same information has more visual impact when subtracted from a sphere (part D and Fig. 5.4a). (**c**) The three-dimensional wire net demonstrates the overall shape of the cornea, but again cannot show the fine detail. However, having obtained the information, it can be subtracted from a sphere (part D) or converted to a slope, curvature or power. (**d**) If a spherical reference plane is used, the local variations in corneal height form a much greater proportion of the overall height represented and are therefore more obvious. The reference sphere has a radius of curvature of 7 mm. Points lying on the reference plane are green; those above are red/yellow, and those below are blue (see Fig. 5.4)

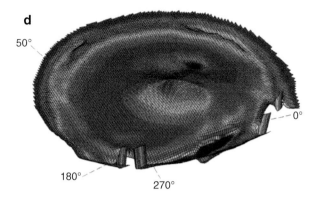

Fig. 5.3 (continued)

equivalent to using a spherical or curved reference surface, rather than a flat reference plane. On the resulting map, local variations in corneal height form a much greater proportion of the overall height represented and are therefore more obvious (Figs. 5.3d and 5.4c). A similar technique can be applied to curvature and power maps [8–10].

Systems using slit photography, or the Scheimpflug principle, are able to measure the shape of the posterior corneal surface and the lens-iris diaphragm and therefore calculate corneal thickness and anterior chamber depth (Fig. 5.4).

Slope and Curvature
Slope and curvature are similar and are both derived from the first differential of height. They represent the "rate of change of height" and as such are a much more sensitive measure of variation in contour across the corneal surface (Fig. 5.5a). Further fine detail of any map can be obtained by using the zoom function (Fig. 5.5b).

Global (axial/sagittal) radius of curvature has spherical bias and is therefore less accurate in the corneal periphery and for irregular surfaces (Fig. 5.6a). In cases where this is important, it is preferable to use local (instantaneous/tangential) radius of curvature (Fig. 5.6b), in which the curvature at each point is calculated with respect to its neighbours (Chap. 1).

Power
Refractive power is a less slightly accurate measure of corneal contour than curvature, especially in abnormal corneas. This is due to the approximations and assumptions made during its derivation (Chap. 1). However, information displayed in this manner is easier to relate to the patient's refractive status and is therefore frequently used in clinical practice (Fig. 5.6).

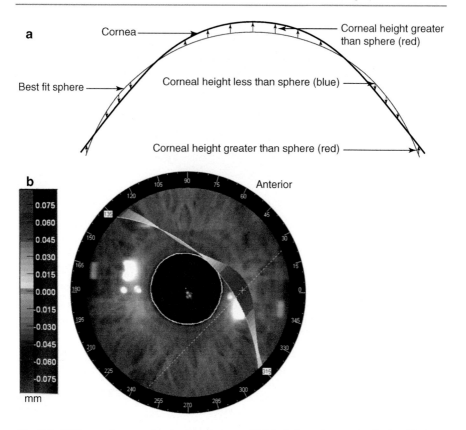

Fig. 5.4 Difference from a sphere and pachymetry. Height information can be depicted in more detail if the information is subtracted from a sphere. In this case of moderate keratoconus, the topography has been derived from slit images. (**a**) The reference plane is spherical. Where the cornea is higher than the sphere (e.g. centrally in a normal prolate cornea), the difference is positive, and colours on the map are warm. Where the cornea is lower than the sphere (e.g. peripherally in a normal cornea), the difference is negative, and the colours are cool. In the very far periphery, the colours become warm again. (**b**) For the anterior elevation map, the green band is the portion of the cornea which is at the same height as a sphere of radius 7.99 mm (42.3D). A cross section through the 135° meridian demonstrates how the cornea is higher than the sphere centrally and lower in the midperiphery. (**c**) The whole anterior elevation map is plotted using the same principles as the cross section in part B. The green band is the portion of the cornea, which is at the same height as the reference sphere (radius 7.99, 42.3D). In keratoconus, the cornea is more prolate than a normal cornea, so the central elevation is more marked. (**d**) Slits can be used to image the posterior corneal surface and reconstruct its topography. In a similar manner to part C, the results have been expressed as the difference in elevation from a sphere (6.59 mm radius of curvature, 51.2D). The posterior cornea is higher than the sphere centrally and lower in the midperiphery. (**e**) The width of the slit gives the thickness of the cornea. The normal cornea is thinner in the centre than the periphery, and this is accentuated in keratoconus. At the thinnest point, marked by the cross, the pachymetry is 403 μ. (**f**) A slit beam also allows the lens-iris diaphragm to be imaged and its anterior surface to be reconstructed. This map shows the depth of the anterior chamber, which is the difference in height between the posterior corneal surface and the lens-iris diaphragm. The anterior chamber is shallowest peripherally and deepest within the pupil margin. (**g**) A sagittal map gives a cross section through the cornea, anterior chamber and the anterior surface of the lens-iris diaphragm

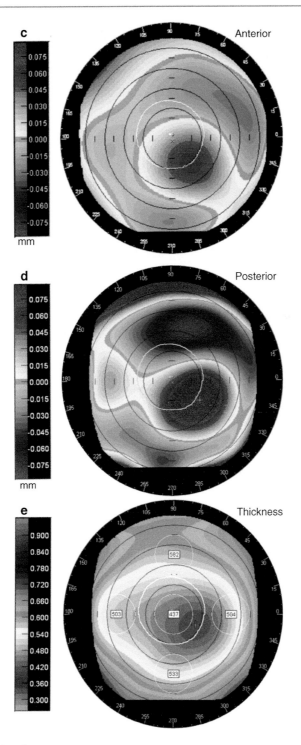

Fig. 5.4 (continued)

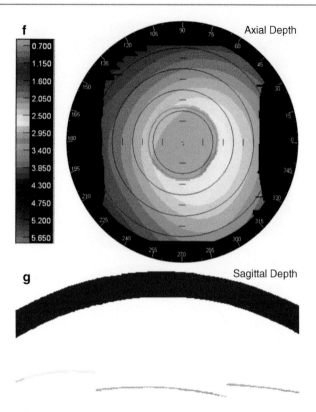

Fig. 5.4 (continued)

Displays

The first computerised display of the corneal surface was by a three-dimensional wire mesh representation, from which only relatively gross distortion could be appreciated [3, 6]. The sensitivity of this technique was improved by presenting the deviation of the corneal shape from spherical [7, 8] or from an idealised corneal shape [2, 10].

The clinical utility of topography increased hugely with the development of two-dimensional colour-coded contour mapping. Today this remains the most frequently used means of representing information derived from Scheimpflug cameras, video-keratoscopes and other topographic devices. Using the computer software, maps can be manipulated and augmented to maximise the information obtained from them. This can be further enhanced by statistical analysis.

Two-Dimensional Maps

In a colour-coded contour map, the corneal surface is represented in two dimensions (x and y), and the third dimension (height/curvature/power of the cornea) is encoded in the colour scheme [2, 4, 11–14]. Areas with the same height/curvature/

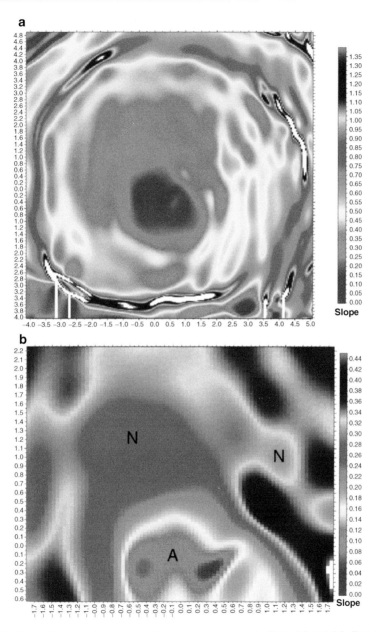

Fig. 5.5 Slope. The same left eye with keratoconus as shown in Figs. 5.2 and 5.3. True height topography was measured by moiré interference, and from it slope was calculated. Slope is the rate of change of height and is therefore a more sensitive way of depicting topography than slope itself. (**a**) The low power view shows that slope is zero (horizontal, red) over the apex of the cone and then becomes increasingly vertical (yellow/green) towards the corneal periphery. The slope is most vertical (blue) at the base of the cone. It is the transition between this vertical area and the more horizontal periphery that iron deposition occurs, producing a Fleischer ring. (**b**) A high-powered view of the central cornea demonstrates how sensitive slope is to corneal irregularities. The two proud nebulae (N) just above the apex (A) of the cone greatly distort the videokeratos-copy mires (Fig 5.2a) but have been reconstructed using this projection-based system

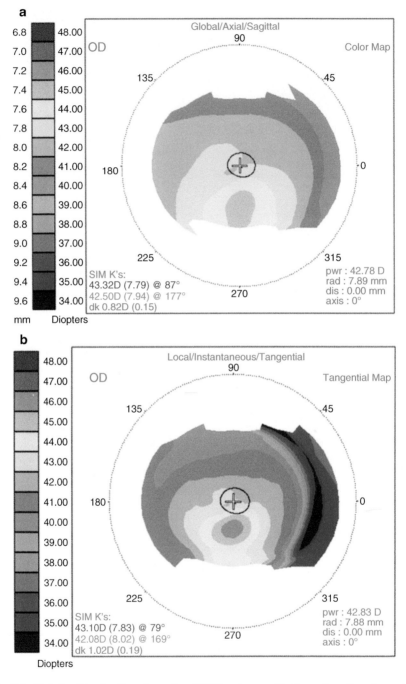

Fig. 5.6 Global and local radius of curvature (ROC) and power. For the scale, radius of curvature or power can be selected. One is converted to the other using the standard keratometry index. (**a**) Global/axial/sagittal/measurements are made relative to the visual axis and therefore have a spherical bias. (**b**) The same map expressed in terms of local/instantaneous/tangential measurements is more accurate over irregularities and in the corneal periphery. In this case of keratoconus, the steep portion of the cone is better localised

power are on the same contour and are therefore depicted in the same colour (Figs. 5.3, 5.4, 5.5 and 5.6). These maps are used most commonly to display topographic information.

Colours

Colour-coded contour maps were initially developed for videokeratoscopy. On these maps, the warmer colours (red, orange, yellow) represented the steeper areas, whereas the cooler colours (green and blue) mark the flatter ones (Table 5.2).

With the introduction of projection-based, slit-photography and Scheimpflug camera-based topography systems, a similar colour-coded system was applied to height maps. For these, the warm colours depicted the high areas, and the low areas are depicted by the cool colours.

As a result, it is extremely important to check the type of scale on the map being studied. For example, in a case of keratoconus, the red area on a height map corresponds to the highest point, which is the apex of the cone. In the same case, the red area on a curvature or power map is the steepest area, which is usually on the side of the cone inferiorly. This becomes obvious when walking up a hill: the steepest part is when walking up the side of the hill. Once the top is reached, it flattens off, and walking becomes easier, although this is the highest part.

Scales

The label on the scale gives the type of measurement which is being displayed: height in mm or μm, slope with no units (or mm/mm) and curvature in mm or power in dioptres.

The appearance of the scale, and therefore the map, is dependent upon the number of steps, the interval between the steps, and the range covered. The first two variables determine the extent of the range. It is therefore essential to check the step interval on the scale before studying the map (Fig. 5.7).

Most systems enable the operator to select between a standardised/absolute scale which is the same for all subjects and a number of variable scales which can be

Table 5.2 Colour coding used for absolute scale maps of videokeratoscopes

Population	Slope	Curvature (mm)	Power (D)	Colour
+3 SD	Steep	7.0	48.0	Red
+1 SD		7.5	45.0	Orange/yellow
Mean	Average	7.8	43.5	Yellow/green
−1 SD		8.0	42.0	Green/light blue
−3 SD	Flat	8.7	39.0	Blue

This is based upon the distribution of corneal curvatures within the population. Average curvatures are coloured yellow or green (depending upon the commercial device). Steeper areas are depicted in warmer colours and flatter areas in cooler colours
SD standard deviation

tailored to the particular case. The selection of the best scale for a given case is determined by the indication for the examination and the particular features to be demonstrated (Table 5.3).

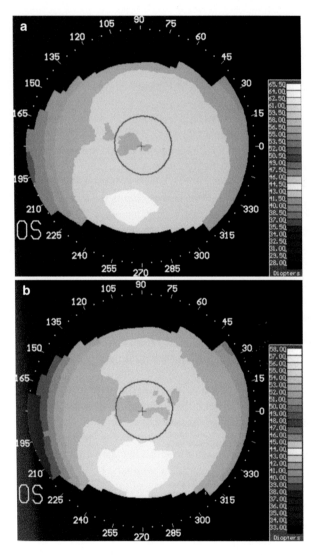

Fig. 5.7 Scale step interval. A case of subclinical keratoconus plotted using scales with different step intervals. (**a**) Absolute scale with a 1.5D step interval. This cornea could be passed as normal, particularly if the scale had not been checked. (**b**) Adjustable scale map with a 1D step interval. The area of inferior steepening becomes obvious. (**c**) 0.5D step interval. (**d**) 0.2D step interval. If this map was studied without reference to the scale, an erroneous diagnosis of severe keratoconus could be made

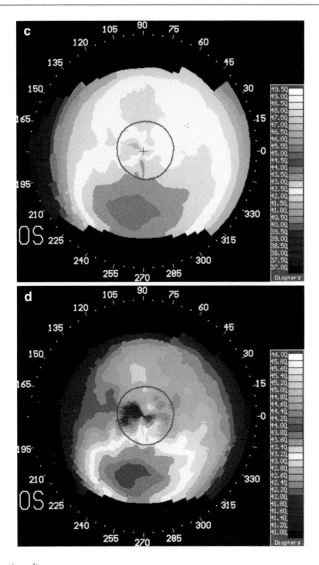

Fig. 5.7 (continued)

Absolute/Standardised Scale

An absolute scale map is one in which there is a fixed colour-coding system: the same colours always represent the same curvatures or powers. This facilitates comparison of the same eye from one occasion to the next, the two eyes of one patient or different patients.

However, there has so far been no standardisation of scales between commercial companies. This makes it more difficult to compare examinations performed using different systems. Given the problems, which occurred in developing standards in

Table 5.3 Comparison of the different types of scales

Standardised/absolute scales	Normalised/relative and customised scales
Standardised	Non-standardised
Good for comparison of maps	Comparison of maps difficult
Large steps	Small steps possible
Low resolution	High resolution
Large range of corneal powers	Narrow range of corneal powers
Good for screening	Subtle features apparent
Good for gross pathology	Good for detail

electrophysiology and perimetry [15], it has long been discussed that a standardised format should be internationally agreed [11–14].

The variability between commercial systems is huge. For example, 1 system uses 34 steps of 0.5D, covering a range of 35–52D. Another system uses 26 steps, which have a 1.5D interval in the range 35.5–50.5D, above and below which 5D steps are used to cover the range 9.0–100D [11].

The allocation of colours on an absolute scale is related to the distribution of corneal powers in the normal population (Table 5.2). Central corneal power has an approximately Gaussian distribution (represented by a bell-shaped curve). The mean central corneal power is 43.50D, which is depicted by a colour from the middle of the spectrum. Approximately 66% of the population have a central corneal power within one standard deviation (± 1 SD) of the mean (42–45D), and this is represented by the adjacent colours on the scale. Less than 3% of the population have a central corneal power beyond ±3 SD, represented by red and dark blue. If these colours are present on an absolute scale map, the cornea is unlikely to be normal.

Normalised/Relative Scale

A normalised scale map uses a set number of colours which are automatically adjusted to fill the range of dioptric values for that single map. The mean power for that cornea is positioned in the centre of the scale.

The normalised scale has the advantage over the absolute scale of using narrower steps between the contours, which provides more detail. Some systems limit how small the steps can be so that the information generated is still clinically relevant (see under section "Adjustable Scale").

However, as the scale may be different for almost every examination, it should be checked carefully before studying the map. For example, the use of a normalised scale can produce a pair of maps of similar appearance for a patient with advanced keratoconus in one eye (using a large step interval) and a subclinical cone in the other eye (using a small step interval).

Adjustable Scale

The adjustable scale map enables the operator to select the step interval and dioptric range of the contours so the topographic information can be displayed to optimum effect. If the same scale is selected for pairs of maps, they may be compared.

Figure 5.7 demonstrates the effect of varying the step interval on the appearance of a map. If a large step interval is used, the range covered is greater, but subtle details may be missed. This is most appropriate for screening or for mapping gross corneal pathology. In contrast, if a very narrow step interval is used, it may highlight small surface irregularities which are not clinically relevant. The most useful step intervals in clinical practice are 1.0 and 1.5D and occasionally 0.5D.

Overlays

Various overlays can be added to topography maps to provide more information and aid interpretation (Table 5.4). Many of these are standardised, but some systems now allow the freehand addition of symbols and text.

Semitransparent Map

Superimposition of a semitransparent topographic map upon the photokeratoscope image of the cornea shows the spatial relationship between the reflected rings and the reconstruction (Fig. 5.8). Focal irregularities due to corneal pathology or tear film disturbance can be matched to the map. The alignment of the cone relative to the cornea can also be confirmed. Poor alignment can lead to the erroneous diagnosis of astigmatism, keratoconus or decentration of a refractive procedure.

Pupil

Graphical markers can be overlaid upon topography maps to provide further information.

Table 5.4 Overlays which can be added to topography maps to provide more information

Overlays	Form	Applications
Pupil margin	Circle	Visually important region
		Pupillary size
		Centration of refractive surgery
Square grid	1 × 1 mm squares	Size, area, location of abnormalities
Polar grid	Axes at 15° intervals	Axis of abnormalities
Optical zones	3, 5, 7 mm rings	Refractive surgery

Fig. 5.8 Semitransparent map. Superimposition of the colour map on the videokeratograph shows how the topography relates to the whole cornea or focal irregularities and enables alignment to be checked. The same map of an eye after PRK is shown in different formats in Figs. 5.10, 5.15 and 5.16

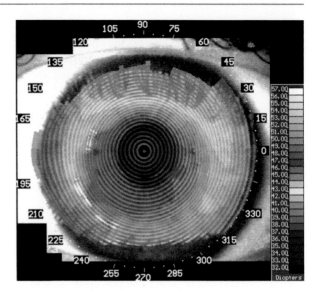

The pupil margin outlines the corneal area of greatest optical importance (Fig. 5.9). The iris acts as a stop, so irregularities within the pupil margin have a greater effect on vision than those outside it.

In addition, the Stiles-Crawford effect operates to minimise the visual impact of aberrations arising from light passing through the peripheral cornea. It is the result of retinal cones being much more sensitive to light which enters the eye paraxially than to light entering obliquely through the peripheral cornea. An overlay can be superimposed upon a topography map to demonstrate the relative importance of different parts of the cornea in the formation of the retinal image. The peripheral cornea is shaded darker, leaving the bright colours at the centre, which is optically more important (Fig. 5.9).

The size and centration of the pupil vary with the level of background illumination. However, if this is standardised while the examination is performed, the identification of abnormally large pupils may help with the planning of the diameter of the optical zone in refractive surgery. The relative position of the pupillary centre and the centre of a treatment zone is a rough guide to whether a refractive procedure is likely to have been decentred.

Grids

The square grid is composed of horizontal and vertical lines 1 mm apart (Fig. 5.10). It is particularly useful for estimating the size, area or position of features, such as a corneal scar. The polar grid gives the axis of abnormalities such as irregular astigmatism or radial keratotomy scars.

Fig. 5.9 Pupil and Stiles-Crawford effect. The importance of different parts of the cornea to its optical effect can be determined in two ways. (**a**) Adding the pupillary overlay encircles the area of the cornea that makes the greatest contribution. (**b**) The Stiles-Crawford facility shades more darkly those peripheral areas of the cornea which contribute least to the retinal image

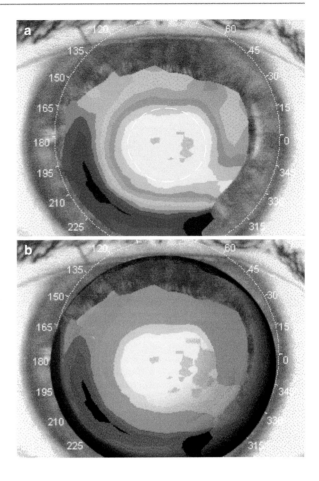

Optical Zones

The optical zones are rings 3 mm, 5 mm and 7 mm in diameter. They can be valuable in refractive surgery for planning procedures or assessing results. They also demonstrate the area of the cornea anterior to the pupillary aperture when the pupil is of different sizes.

Axes

An axis is the meridian of either greatest or least slope. They may be calculated for the cornea as a whole (orthogonal), for a couple of separate zones (zonal) or individually for each diameter (each ring in the case of videokeratoscopes) (Table 5.5). The derivation of these values will be described for videokeratoscopy, although the method can be applied to data obtained by other techniques.

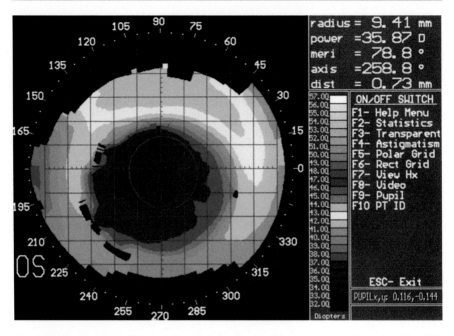

Fig. 5.10 Square grid and cursor. Overlying a square grid shows that the diameter of the PRK treatment zone is 6 mm. The coordinates of the centre of the pupil are given in the bottom right corner. The cursor has been moved to the centre of the treatment zone, and the parameters of this point are given in the cursor box in the top right corner. This shows that the treatment is displaced from the visual axis by a distance of 0.73 mm along an axis of 259°. The box on the right lists some of the other display options

Table 5.5 Astigmatic axes which can be added to a corneal topography map to provide additional information

Axes	Derivation	Applications
Orthogonal	Meridian with greatest mean power in central 3 mm zone and the axis at 90° to it	Equivalent to the keratometer
		Only of use in regular astigmatism
Zonal	Steepest and flattest axes in the 3 mm, 5 mm and 7 mm zones	Data provided in statistical indices box
Instantaneous	Continuous lines joining points of maximum power or minimum power on each ring	"True axes"
		Useful in irregular astigmatism

Their derivation is described for videokeratoscopes, although similar techniques can be applied to topography obtained by other techniques

Orthogonal Axes

The orthogonal axes represent the major and minor meridians (Fig. 5.11a). They are determined by averaging the power from the rings within the central 3 mm zone along every meridian. The major axis is that meridian with the greater average power. The minor meridian lies at right angles to the major meridian, and is not necessarily that with the lowest average power.

These axes simulate those measured by the keratometer. As such, they provide a limited amount of information.

Zonal Axes

The zonal axes are the steepest and flattest meridian within the 3 mm, 5 mm and 7 mm zones (Fig. 5.11b). The statistical indices box displays the numerical values for power (dioptres), radius of curvature (mm) and axis (degrees) for each of the four axes, in each of the three zones.

Instantaneous Axes

The instantaneous axes are the true major and minor axes (Fig. 5.11c). They are continuous lines joining points of maximum or minimum power on each ring. The information they provide is more detailed than that given by the orthogonal or zonal axes and demonstrates that axes are not necessarily radial or perpendicular.

Three-Dimensional Representations

Three-Dimensional Wire Net

The three-dimensional wire net was one of the earliest ways in which corneal topography was represented. Current computer software can formulate these representations relatively easily to provide visual impact, but they have the disadvantage of only demonstrating relatively gross irregularities of the corneal surface (Fig. 5.3c). A more sensitive way of using three-dimensional nets is to plot the difference from a sphere of known size [7, 8] or from an idealised corneal shape [10]. However, most systems rely upon two-dimensional maps and cross sections to provide clinically relevant information.

Cross Sections

Height Cross Sections

Cross sections only contain data from one axis, but they are a very sensitive way of displaying local irregularities. Plotting two cross sections simultaneously enhances this: one from a relatively normal axis and one from an affected axis (Figs. 5.3a and 5.12).

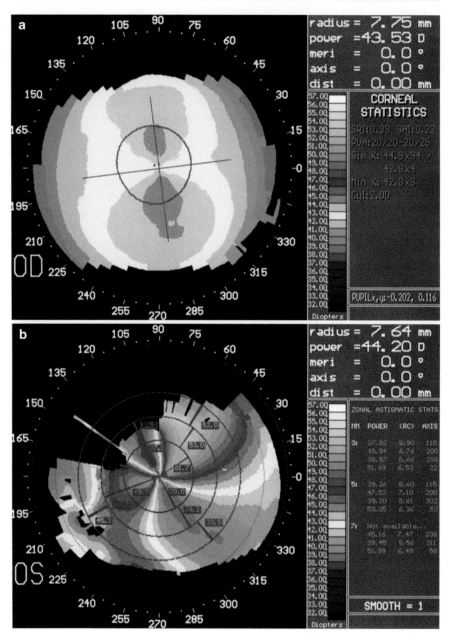

Fig. 5.11 Astigmatic axes. (**a**) Orthogonal axes are suitable for regular astigmatism to show the spherocylindrical keratometry of the central 3 mm in the major (steepest) axis and in the minor axis 90° to it. (**b**) Zonal axes show the steepest and flattest meridian within the 3 mm, 5 mm and 7 mm zones, the numerical values of which are displayed in the statistics box on the right. The irregularity of this postkeratoplasty astigmatism is shown by the variation in the position of the steepest and flattest meridian in the different zones. (**c**) Instantaneous axes join the points of maximum or minimum power on each ring. In this case of peripheral guttering, the axes are neither radial nor orthogonal. Good vision would not be achieved by a spherocylindrical spectacle prescription. The left eye of the same patient is shown in Fig. 9.5

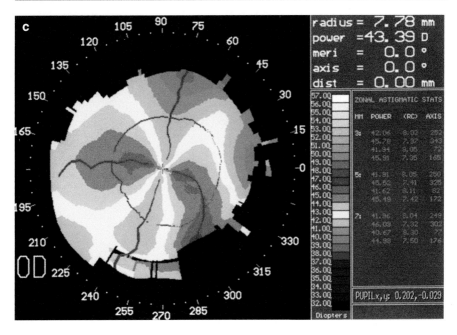

Fig. 5.11 (continued)

Refraction Profile

The refraction profile is the power of the cornea in the major and minor axes plotted against the zone diameter (Fig. 5.13). The difference between the two axes is the astigmatism.

Isometric Map

On an isometric map, the rings are straightened into lines from 0 to 360° (Fig. 5.14). The dioptric power of each point on a ring is plotted against the axis on which it lies. Isometric maps are displayed both two dimensional, when the lines appear superimposed as if viewed from the side, and three dimensional, when the lines are spread out, as if viewed from a higher point. The straighter the lines, the more spherical the cornea. This is particularly useful for determining whether astigmatism is regular and quantifying how it changes over time [16].

Multiple Displays

Serial Maps

Many devices provide an option of displaying two to six maps simultaneously. However, each map is usually smaller than in the single displays, resulting in a loss of detail. When making comparisons, it is important that the scale of the maps is the same.

Fig. 5.12 Height cross section. In this patient with a peripheral corneal gutter (map in Fig. 8.4), plotting both the affected axis (90°, red) and the unaffected axis (180°, black) demonstrated that the gutter was 1.25 mm wide and 175 μm deep

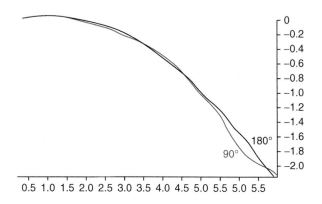

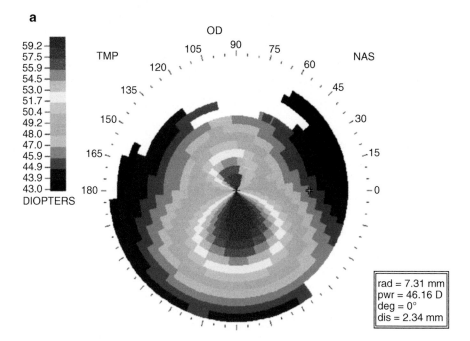

Fig. 5.13 Refraction profile. (**a**) The colour map shows moderate keratoconus. (**b**) The refraction profile plots the dioptric power across the corneal diameter in the steepest (red) and flattest (blue) meridia. The temporal and nasal portions of the cornea (blue line) are relatively symmetric and show the normal degree of flattening from the centre to the periphery. The inferior cornea is steeper than the superior cornea (red line), as is typical of keratoconus. The astigmatism (green line) is the difference in power between the steepest and flattest meridian at a given distance from the corneal centre (note the inversion of the axis: greater astigmatism is shown lower down)

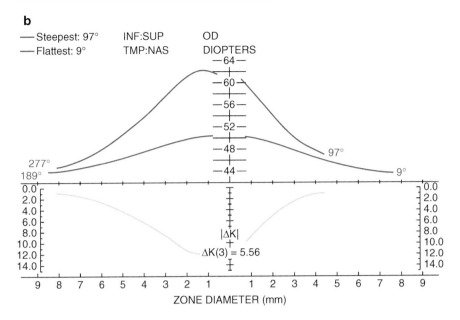

b

— Steepest: 97° INF:SUP OD
— Flattest: 9° TMP:NAS DIOPTERS

$|\Delta K|$
$\Delta K(3) = 5.56$

ZONE DIAMETER (mm)

Fig. 5.13 (continued)

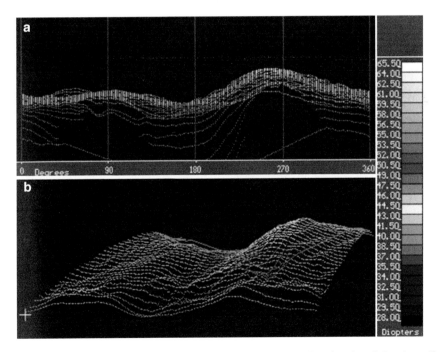

Fig. 5.14 Isometric map. The power of the points on each ring are plotted against their axis, as if the rings have been straightened out. The colour map for this case of mild keratoconus is shown in Fig. 5.7. (**a**) Two-dimensional view showing that the cornea is steepest in the 270° meridian. (**b**) Three-dimensional view showing that the steepening is greatest nearer the centre (at the front of the graph) than in the periphery (towards the back of the graph)

Difference Maps

A difference map represents the change in corneal contour from one time point to another. It is calculated by subtracting the first map from the second [17] (Fig. 5.15). This is useful for demonstrating the change occurring as a result of a surgical procedure or during the subsequent healing phase. However, the reliability of such maps is dependent upon the accurate alignment of the equipment whilst both images were obtained [18].

Fourier analysis of a difference map can separate the four different components of change: spherical, skewness, regular astigmatism and residual astigmatism [19]. This enables each aspect of the induced change to be analysed separately.

Some systems contain software which plots the difference between a measured map and the ideal aspheric cornea [9]. The ideal cornea for an individual is calculated using the measured central corneal power for that individual and an asphericity index of −0.26. The difference map generated demonstrates how the contour of the cornea differs from normal and is particularly useful for diagnosing corneal diseases, such as keratoconus, in which the cornea changes its overall shape.

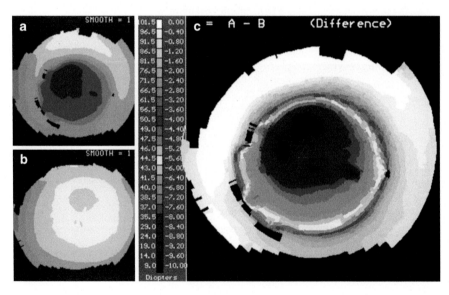

Fig. 5.15 Difference map. Following PRK, subtraction of (**a**) the map taken at week 1 postoperatively from (**b**) the preoperative map gives (**c**) the change in topography which has occurred as a result of the treatment. There has been no significant change outside the treatment zone and maximal change at the centre of the treatment zone

Tailored Displays

To facilitate the application of corneal topography in clinical practice, some systems provide the option of multiple displays containing the elements most pertinent to a particular clinical activity [20]. For example, a display tailored to the diagnosis of corneal pathology contains a standardised map, normalised map, profile difference map, distortion map and indices relating to astigmatism, the pupil and predicted visual function [9]. A tailored display for incisional refractive surgery contains maps of the anterior and posterior corneal elevation, axial power and pachymetry and indices relating to the astigmatism in different zones. Some software contains nomograms which can calculate the site and depth of the incisions required. Displays specific to contact lens fitting are described in Chap. 7.

Numeric and Statistical Displays

Numbers can be used to provide topographic information in two ways. Firstly, the actual measurements can be listed for a small number of points (e.g. in the cursor box or numeric maps). Secondly, statistical analysis can generate numbers which summarise a particular feature of the whole cornea.

Numbers have the advantage that they are amenable to further statistical analysis. This is important when studying groups of patients or making objective comparisons. However, their disadvantage is that they ignore much of the available data, and as a result, detailed topographic information is lost.

Cursor Box

The cursor is a movable point marker. Its initial or default position is at the corneal reflex centre (the corneal apex). The mouse or arrow keys can then be used to move it to any other position on the map (Figs. 5.1 and 5.10).

The cursor box provides information about the cornea at the single point over which the cursor lies (Table 5.6). This includes its radius of curvature and power and its distance and axis from the corneal reflex centre or the entrance pupil centre (Chap. 6).

In this way the cursor may be used to provide information about an area of interest, such as the steepest portion of a cone. It can also be used to measure distances, such as the decentration of a refractive treatment zone.

Table 5.6 Information
displayed in the cursor box

Cursor box
Corneal data at site of cursor
Radius of curvature (mm)
Dioptric power (D)
Position of cursor from videokeratoscope centre and/or entrance pupil centre
Axis (°)
Distance (mm)

Numeric Map

The numeric map gives about ten numeric values (dioptres or mm curvature) along 8–16 meridians (Fig. 5.16). This replaces the need to refer to the scale when determining the contour of a certain point or when comparing two maps [21]. For groups of corneas, the topography of discrete regions can be represented numerically to make the data amenable to statistical methods [22–24].

Statistical Indices

Statistical indices (parameters/quantitative descriptors) (Table 5.7) are numbers, which summarise a particular feature of the cornea [25–27] (Figs. 5.1, 5.10 and 5.16). These can then be compared to a normal range or grouped to summarise the topography of several patients, as in clinical trials. Different commercial systems may give indices different names, but they are calculated in a similar way and perform the same functions.

Simulated Keratometry Readings

The simulated keratometry readings (SimK) provide information equivalent to that measured by the keratometer and are therefore primarily for historical reference. They are calculated by determining the average power along each meridian in the central (within the 3 mm zone) or paracentral (rings 7–9) area. The major axis is that with the greatest power, and the minor axis is at 90° to it. Alternatively, the minimum keratometry reading (Min K) can be calculated, which is the meridian with the lowest mean power. The cylinder is the difference between the major and minor axes. These readings have the same limitations as keratometry [28].

Sphero-Equivalent Power

The sphero-equivalent power (SEP) is the effective refractive power of the cornea within the 3 mm pupil zone, taking into account the Stiles-Crawford effect. It is calculated using data from all meridians. For corneas with irregular astigmatism, it is more reliable than keratometry for the calculation of the power of an intraocular lens.

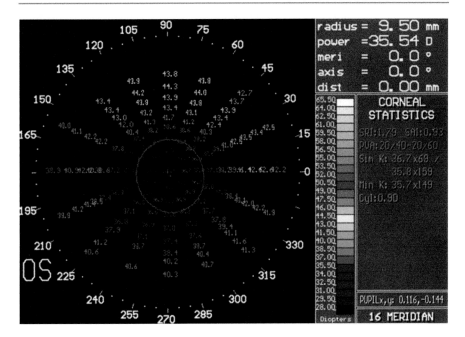

Fig. 5.16 Numeric map and statistical indices. The colour map of this case of PRK is shown in Fig. 5.10. This numeric map gives that actual value of the power at about 100 corneal locations. This may be useful when analysing the data from groups of patients. The surface regularity index (SRI) is elevated due to the rapid changes in power which occur between adjacent points, particularly towards the edge of the treatment zone. The surface asymmetry index (SAI) is elevated because the treatment is slightly decentred, resulting in differences in power between opposite points. As a result of this irregularity, the potential visual acuity (PVA) reduced. The simulated keratometry readings (SimK) give the paracentral power in the steepest axis and at 90° to it, whereas the minimum keratometry reading is taken from the flattest index. These values are also shown in red because they are abnormally flat due to the treatment. The astigmatism (cyl) is the difference between the SimK values

Asphericity

In the conic equation describing the shape of the normal cornea, the value for asphericity (Q) is −0.26. If the cornea is flatter than normal in the midperiphery, Q will be more negative. If it is steeper than normal in the midperiphery, as after radial keratotomy, Q will be less negative or even positive [9, 29–32].

Surface Asymmetry Index

The surface asymmetry index (SAI) is a measure of the difference in corneal powers between points on the same ring 180° apart. This is calculated from over the entire corneal surface, although the central points are given more weighting. The power distribution across a normal corneal surface is fairly symmetrical (SAI <0.5). Therefore the SAI can be a useful quantitative indicator of the

Table 5.7 Statistical indices presented in topographic displays

Statistical index/ parameter	Description	Application
Simulated keratometry readings (SimK)	Axis of greatest power in the central cornea and the axis at 90° to it	Comparison with keratometer readings limited
Sphero-equivalent power (SEP)	Effective refractive power within 3 mm zone	Calculation of IOL power in irregular astigmatism
Asphericity (Q)	Flattening or steepening of midperiphery	Optical aberrations following refractive surgery
Surface asymmetry index (SAI)	Difference between opposite semimeridians	Progression of corneal disease
Inferior-superior value (I-SV)	Power difference between superior and inferior cornea	Differentiation of keratoconus from normal corneas
Keratoconus prediction index (KPI)	Derived from eight other indices	Detection of keratoconus and differentiation from other corneal disease
Surface regularity index (SRI)	Local variations in corneal contour	Detection of irregular astigmatism
Corneal uniformity index (CUI)		
Root-mean-square deviation (RMS)		
Potential visual acuity (PVA)	Range of acuity expected, based on topography alone; correlated with SRI	Effect of irregular astigmatism on acuity
Predicted corneal acuity (PCA)		

Similar indices are used by different commercial devices but may be given different names

progression of corneal diseases such as keratoconus or peripheral corneal gutters [26, 33].

Inferior-Superior Value
The inferior-superior value (I-SV) is a method similar to the SAI designed to differentiate keratoconus from normal corneas [34]. It is calculated from the refractive power difference between five inferior points and five superior points 3 mm from the centre at 30° intervals.

Keratoconus Prediction Index
The keratoconus prediction index (KPI) is a much more specific but more complex index derived from the SimK, SAI and five other indices [35, 36], (Table 10.2).

Surface Regularity Index
The surface regularity index (SRI) is a measure of the local regularity of the corneal surface within the central 4.5 mm diameter. Within this area, the power of each point is compared with that of the points immediately surrounding it. This

index correlates well with visual function. Normal corneas have low SRI values (SRI < 1.0), whereas those with poor visual potential due to irregular astigmatism have high values. A similar measure is the corneal uniformity index (CUI), which varies from 0% if the cornea is completely irregular to 100% if it is completely uniform. In systems measuring corneal height, surface smoothness can be calculated from the root-mean-square (RMS) deviation from the best-fit surface [37].

Potential Visual Acuity

The potential visual acuity (PVA) or predicted corneal acuity (PCA) is the estimated range of visual acuity which could be expected, if the cornea was the only factor-limiting vision. Corneas with irregular astigmatism have lower potential acuities.

Optical Aberrations

The eye has significant optical aberrations [38–40], which may be altered by corneal refractive procedures [41].

Ray-tracing techniques and corneal modulation transfer functions can be applied to corneal topography maps to estimate the severity of various optical aberrations generated, including spherical, chromatic and coma [42, 43]. Wavefront aberrometry has enabled a greater understanding of these optical imperfections and improved outcomes following laser refractive surgery (see Chaps. 13 and 14).

Interpretation

Application of Basic Principles

Any topography map can be interpreted if it is approached systematically and the basic principles are applied.

Pattern Recognition

With experience, pattern recognition contributes to the interpretation of maps, which as a result becomes faster. However, before studying the topography of corneas with pathology or which have undergone surgery, it is most important to be familiar with the appearance of normal corneas (Chap. 6). Also it is necessary to be able to distinguish between those abnormalities on the maps which are due to artefact and those arising from the cornea itself.

To aid the description and comparison of topographic maps, several authors have devised classifications for the patterns typical of normal corneas and those occurring in corneal disease or as a result of surgery. These are described in the *relevant chapters*. Although there is high concordance between individuals classifying maps, it would be more objective for a computer to assign maps to the appropriate category.

Neural Networks

In other fields, such as the analysis of fundus photographs in diabetic retinopathy, significant progress has been made with artificial intelligence (AI) and its ability to recognise disease patterns. In a recent study by Gulshan et al., researchers assessed 9963 images from 4997 patients to train a computer to recognize diabetic retinopathy. The computer achieved 97.5% sensitivity and 93.4% specificity [44]. Similar programs are under development in glaucoma screening. Given the relative simplicity of the images generated by corneal topography compared to those of the fundus, similar rapid progress may be seen in this field [45].

Artificial neural networks are composed of many similar elements, akin to neurons, which are multiply interconnected by electronic or optical links, corresponding to axons and dendrites with synapses [46]. As information passes through the network, it modifies the electronic or optical properties of the semiconductor components, thereby altering the ease with which later information can traverse the same pathway. This process is termed "Deep Learning". Most learning algorithms would require a very large number of training cycles, in which a topography map is presented to the computer and its classification entered. A recent study has shown that a deep learning AI algorithm was as accurate in detecting skin cancer as board-certified dermatologists [47].

Further development of this technology will require a greater knowledge of the operation of large complex networks, either from observation of the nervous system and the way it functions or from theoretical models.

References

*References Particularly Worth Reading

1. Cairns G, McGhee CN. Orbscan computerized topography: attributes, applications, and limitations. J Cataract Refract Surg. 2005;31(1):205–20.
2. Belin MW, Khachikian SS. An introduction to understanding elevation-based topography: how elevation data are displayed – a review. Clin Exp Ophthalmol. 2009;37(1):14–29.
3. Klyce SD. Computer-assisted corneal topography: high resolution graphic presentation and analysis of keratoscopy. Invest Ophthalmol Vis Sci. 1984;25:1426–35.
4. Maguire LJ, Singer DE, Klyce SD. Graphic presentation of computer analysed keratoscope photographs. Arch Ophthalmol. 1987;105:223–30.
5. *Corbett MC, O'Brart DPS, Stultiens BATh, Jongsma FHM, Marshall J. Corneal topography using a new moiré image-based system. Eur J Implant Refract Surg. 1995;7:353–70.
6. Young JA, Siegel IM. Isomorphic corneal topography: a clinical approach to 3-D representation of the corneal surface. Refract Corneal Surg. 1993;9:74–8.
7. Warnicki JW, Rehkopf PG, Curtin DY, Burns SA, Arffa RC, Stuart JC. Corneal topography using computer analyzed rasterstereographic images. Appl Opt. 1988;27:1135–40.
8. Young JA, Siegel IM. Three-dimensional digital subtraction modeling of corneal topography. J Refract Surg. 1995;11:188–93.
9. *Holladay JT. Corneal topography using the Holladay diagnostic summary. J Cataract Refract Surg. 1997;23:209–21.

10. Huber C, Huber A, Gruber H. Three-dimensional representations of corneal deformations from keratotopographic data. J Cataract Refract Surg. 1997;23:202–8.
11. *Wilson SE, Klyce SD, Husseini ZM. Standardized color-coded maps for corneal topography. Ophthalmology. 1993;100:1723–7.
12. Siegel IM. Standardized color-coded corneal maps [letter]. Ophthalmology. 1994;101:795.
13. Gailitis RP, Lipsitt KL. Standardized color-coded corneal maps [letter]. Ophthalmology. 1994;101:795–6.
14. Wilson SE, Klyce SD. Standardized color-coded corneal maps [reply]. Ophthalmology. 1994;101:796–7.
15. Suzuki Y, Araie M, Ohashi Y. Sectorization of the central 30° visual field in glaucoma. Ophthalmology. 1993;100:69–75.
16. Friedman NE, Zadnik K, Mutti DO, Fusaro RE. Quantifying corneal toricity from videokeratography with Fourier analysis. J Refract Surg. 1996;12:108–13.
17. Holladay JT, Cravy TV, Koch DD. Calculation of surgically induced refractive change following ocular surgery. J Cataract Refract Surg. 1992;18:429–43.
18. Johnson DA, Haight DH, Kelly SE, Muller J, Swinger CA, Tostanoski J, Odrich MG. Reproducibility of videokeratographic digital subtraction maps after excimer laser photorefractive keratectomy. Ophthalmology. 1996;103:1392–8.
19. Olsen T, Dam-Johansen M, Beke T, Hjortdal JO. Evaluating surgically induced astigmatism by Fourier analysis of corneal topography data. J Cataract Refract Surg. 1996;22:318–23.
20. Grimm BB. Communicating with keratography. J Refract Surg. 1996;12:156–9.
21. Rowsey JJ, Reynolds AE, Brown DR. Corneal topography. Corneascope. Arch Ophthalmol. 1981;99:1093–100.
22. *Vass C, Menapace R. Computerised statistical analysis of corneal topography for the evaluation of changes in corneal shape after surgery. Am J Ophthalmol. 1994;118:177–84.
23. Vass C, Menapace R, Rainer G, Schulz H. Improved algorithm for statistical batch-by-batch analysis of corneal topographic data. J Cataract Refract Surg. 1997;23:903–12.
24. Vass C, Menapace R, Amon M, Hirsch U, Yousef A. Batch-by-batch analysis of topographic changes induced by sutured and sutureless clear corneal incisions. J Cataract Refract Surg. 1996;22:324–30.
25. Dingeldein SA, Klyce SD, Wilson SE. Quantitative descriptors of corneal shape derived from the computer-assisted analysis of photokeratographs. Refract Corneal Surg. 1989;5:372–8.
26. *Wilson SE, Klyce SD. Quantitative descriptors of corneal topography. A clinical study. Arch Ophthalmol. 1991;109:349–53.
27. Rabinowitz YS. Videokeratographic indices to aid in screening for keratoconus. J Refract Surg. 1995;11:371–9.
28. Sanders RD, Gills JP, Martin RG. When keratometric measurements do not accurately reflect corneal topography. J Cataract Refract Surg. 1993;19(Suppl):131–5.
29. Fleming JF. Should refractive surgeons worry about corneal asphericity? Refract Corneal Surg. 1990;6:455–7.
30. Eghbali F, Yeung KK, Maloney RK. Topographic determination of corneal asphericity and its lack of effect on the outcome of radial keratotomy. Am J Ophthalmol. 1995;119:275–80.
31. Calossi A. Corneal asphericity and spherical aberration. J Refract Surg. 2007;23(5):505–14.
32. Bottos KM, Leite MT, Aventura-Isidro M, et al. Corneal asphericity and spherical aberration after refractive surgery. J Cataract Refract Surg. 2011;37(6):1109–15.
33. Borderie VM, Laroche L. Measurement of irregular astigmatism using semimeridian data from videokeratographs. J Refract Surg. 1996;12:595–600.
34. Rabinowitz YS, McDonnell PJ. Computer-assisted corneal topography in keratoconus. Refract Corneal Surg. 1989;5:400–8.
35. Madea N, Klyce SD, Smolek MK, Thompson HW. Automated keratoconus screening with corneal topography analysis. Invest Ophthalmol Vis Sci. 1994;35:2749–57.
36. Burns DM, Johnston FM, Frazer DG, et al. Keratoconus: an analysis of corneal asymmetry. Br J Ophthalmol. 2004;88:1252–5.

37. Liang F-Q, Geasey SD, del Cerro M, Aquavella JV. A new procedure for evaluating smooth-ness of corneal surface following 193nm excimer laser ablation. Refract Corneal Surg. 1992;8:459–65.
38. Howland HC, Howland B. A subjective method for the measurement of monochromatic aber-rations of the eye. J Opt Soc Am. 1977;67:1508–18.
39. Walsh G, Charman WN, Howland HC. Objective technique for the determination of mono-chromatic aberrations of the human eye. J Opt Soc Am A. 1984;1:987–92.
40. Liang J, Williams DR. Aberrations and retinal image quality of the normal human eye. J Opt Soc Am A. 1997;14:2873–83.
41. Oshika T, Klyce SD, Applegate RA. Comparison of corneal wavefront aberrations after pho-torefractive keratectomy and laser in situ keratomileusis. Am J Ophthalmol. 1999;127:1–7.
42. Seiler T, Reckmann W, Maloney RK. Effective spherical aberration of the cornea as a quantita-tive descriptor in corneal topography. J Cataract Refract Surg. 1993;19(Suppl):155–65.
43. Oliver KM, Hemenger RP, Corbett MC, O'Brart DPS, Verma S, Marshall J, Tomlinson A. Corneal optical aberrations induced by photorefractive keratectomy. J Refract Surg. 1997;13:246–54.
44. Gulshan V, Peng L, Coram M, et al. Development and validation of a deep learning algorithm for detection of diabetic retinopathy in retinal fundus photographs. JAMA. 2016;316(22):2402–10.
45. *Maeda M, Klyce SD, Smolek MK. Neural network classification of corneal topography. Invest Ophthalmol Vis Sci. 1995;36:1327–35.
46. Psaltis D, Brady D, Gu X-G, Lin S. Holography in artificial neural networks. Nature. 1990;343:325–30.
47. Esteva A, Kuprel B, Novoa RA, et al. Dermatologist-level classification of skin cancer with deep neural networks. Nature. 2017;542(7639):115–8.

Part II

The Normal Cornea

Normal Topography

6

The assessment of corneal topography is a valuable tool in the diagnosis and management of certain corneal conditions. However, before using this technique to diagnose abnormalities of corneal shape, it is vital to have a good understanding of the normal corneal shape and its natural variations. When abnormalities of corneal topography are detected, it is also important to be able to determine whether these are a result of abnormalities of the cornea itself, or whether they are artefacts arising from errors in image acquisition or analysis.

Normal Corneal Shape

Corneal Anatomy and Optics

The cornea has a unique structure, quite unlike that of any other tissue in the body. As a result of its position forming the wall of the anterior portion of the globe, the cornea has to meet strict physical criteria and perform a variety of specialist functions. As part of the tough outer coat of the eye, the cornea, together with the sclera, should maintain the intraocular pressure, support the intraocular structures and resist trauma and infection.

However, in addition to its mechanical function, the cornea has two major roles in vision. Firstly, its anterior surface is the major refractive element of the eye, responsible for bringing an image to a focus. Secondly, it is transparent to enable light to be transmitted to the retina.

Anterior Corneal Surface

The cornea contributes two-thirds of the total refractive power of the eye. The remainder is provided by the lens (Table 6.1). The greatest refractive effect is achieved at the interface between the air and the tear film, as this represents the greatest change in refractive index in the light pathway. The power generated at this interface is determined by its shape, and that is in turn dependent upon the

© Springer Nature Switzerland AG 2019
M. Corbett et al., *Corneal Topography*,
https://doi.org/10.1007/978-3-030-10696-6_6

Table 6.1 Anatomical and optical indices of the normal anterior segment

Anterior segment structures		Average	Range
Refractive index			
Air		1.0	
Cornea		1.376	
	Standard keratometric index (SKI)	*1.337*	
	Corneal epithelium	1.401	
	Anterior corneal stroma	1.380	
	Posterior corneal stroma	1.373	
	Aqueous	1.336	
	Lens	1.38–1.42	
Central radius of curvature			
	Anterior corneal surface	*7.8 mm*	*7.0–8.6 mm*
	Posterior corneal surface	6.7 mm	
Dioptric power			
	Anterior corneal surface	49.50 D	
	Posterior corneal surface	−6.00 D	
	Net corneal power	*43.50 D*	*39–48 D*
	Net lens power	20.00 D	
	Total power of the eye	63.50 D	
Thickness			
	Central cornea	0.56 mm	
	Peripheral cornea	1.20 mm	
	Corneal epithelium	0.06 mm	50–60 μm

The method of converting radius of curvature to power is described in Chap. 1. The standard keratometric index (SKI) is the index used to calculate the net corneal power from the anterior corneal curvature

shape of the underlying anterior corneal surface. In the normal cornea, the average central radius of curvature is 7.8 mm, which contributes a refractive power of 49.50 D.

Posterior Corneal Surface

The posterior corneal surface has a slightly steeper radius of curvature (6.7 mm) than the anterior surface, because the cornea is thicker in the periphery than in the centre. It has a negative power (−6.00D) because light diverges as it passes through a convex surface from a medium of higher refractive index to one of lower refractive index. The posterior surface is less important in refraction, as there is less difference between the refractive indices of the cornea and the aqueous. The combination of the effects of the anterior and posterior corneal surfaces gives an average net central corneal power of 43.50 D.

Net Corneal Power

The net power of a lens system is the sum of the power of its components. For the power of the cornea (P_C, in dioptres), this can be approximated to the sum of the powers of its anterior (P_A) and posterior (P_P) surfaces. As described in Chap. 1, for any surface of radius of curvature r (in metres), bounded by media with refractive indices n_1 and n_2:

$$P = \frac{n_2 - n_1}{r}$$

if: $P_C = P_A + P_P$

$$\text{then } P_C = \frac{n_2 - n_1}{r_A} + \frac{n_3 - n_2}{r_B}$$

For any case, the refractive index of air (n_1) is 1. The anterior corneal curvature (r_A) is measured by corneal topography. However, it is not possible to measure the posterior corneal curvature (r_B) or the refractive index of the cornea (n_2) or the aqueous (n_3). In clinical practice, these three variables are replaced by the standard keratometric index (SKI):

$$P_C = \frac{SKI - 1}{r_A}$$

Therefore, the SKI is a combined estimate of the posterior corneal curvature and the refractive indices of the cornea and the aqueous. In the normal eye, it has a value of 1.3375. Therefore:

$$P_C = 0.3375 / r_A$$

or, if the radius of curvature is expressed in millimetres rather than metres:

$$P_C = 337.5 / R_A \text{ (in mm)}$$

Corneal Asphericity

The central 4 mm of the cornea is approximately spherical. Outside this, the peripheral cornea is aspheric and radially asymmetric: the radius of curvature changes from centre to limbus, and does so at different rates along different semimeridians [1–3]. The profile of a cornea along any meridian can be considered as part of an ellipse [4]. The normal cornea has a prolate shape, as occurs at the narrow end of an ellipse, meaning that it becomes flatter from the centre to the periphery (Fig. 6.1). The reverse pattern is an oblate shape, as occurs on the long side of an ellipse. This is only seen in abnormal corneas, for example, after radial keratotomy [5].

Many authors have tried to describe the complex aspheric asymmetric shape of the normal cornea either mathematically or graphically [6, 7]. However, no method is entirely accurate. In the conic equation, the value Q represents the corneal asphericity [8] (Table 6.2). For a sphere, $Q = 0$. For prolate surfaces (flatter in the periphery) $Q < 0$, and for oblate surfaces $Q > 0$.

The level of sophistication required from any method of representing the corneal surface is dependent upon its potential applications. Fortunately in the routine

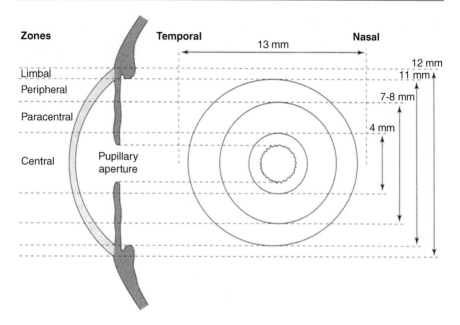

Fig. 6.1 Zones of the cornea. Diagrammatic representation of the right cornea in vertical section (left) and from anteriorly (right). The cornea is horizontally oval and steeper centrally than in the periphery. Its anterior surface can be arbitrarily divided into four zones: central, paracentral, peripheral and limbal

Table 6.2 Corneal asphericity

Asphericity (Q)	Shape	Description	Example
>0	Oblate	Peripheral steepening	Radial keratotomy
0	*Spherical*	*Uniform curvature*	*Steel calibration ball*
<0	Prolate	Peripheral flattening	
−0.26	Prolate	Mild peripheral flattening	Normal cornea
< −0.26	Prolate	Marked peripheral flattening	Keratoconus

The Q value describes the extent to which the cornea becomes steeper or flatter from the centre towards the periphery

clinical setting, it is often sufficient to liken the cornea to a spherocylindrical lens, as proven by the number of optical defects which can be adequately corrected by simple spectacle lenses.

Astigmatism

Astigmatism can be defined as the refractive error in which no point focus is formed owing to the unequal refraction of light in different meridians [9]. It may originate from asymmetry or decentration of the optical surfaces of the eye, or irregularities in refractive index (Table 6.3).

Astigmatism was first recognised by the English scientist Thomas Young in 1801, who described the defect in his own eyes [10]. The optics of the condition

Table 6.3 Astigmatism – definitions, aetiology and types

Astigmatism	
Definition	Refractive error
	No point focus is formed
	Unequal refraction of light by different meridians
Aetiology	Asymmetry in the curvature of the optical surfaces of the eye
	Decentration of optical surfaces of the eye
	Irregularities in the refractive index of the ocular media
Regular astigmatism	Uniform change in power from one meridian to the next
	Major and minor axes perpendicular
Irregular astigmatism	Curvature conforms to no geometric pattern
"With-the-rule" astigmatism	Steeper curvature vertically
	Corrected by negative cylinder at axis 180°
"Against-the-rule" astigmatism	Steeper curve horizontally/corrected by negative cylinder at 90°

were subsequently clarified by Donders [11]. He distinguished between regular and irregular astigmatism. Regular astigmatism is where the refractive power changes gradually from one meridian to the next by uniform increments. Irregular astigmatism is where the changes in the curvature of the meridians conforms to no geometric pattern.

The most common cause of astigmatic error is due to the astigmatic curvature of the anterior corneal surface. This may occur both physiologically and pathologically. The average difference between the refractive powers of the major and minor cornea meridians usually lies between 0.50 and 1.00D. In about 90% of eyes, the meridian of greatest curvature is within 30° of the vertical meridian [1]. This is termed "direct" or "with-the-rule" astigmatism. This physiological tendency for the cornea to have a steeper curvature vertically has not been adequately explained [12]. It is usually neutralised by inverse astigmatism in the posterior corneal surface or the lens.

Zones of the Corneal Surface

Classically, the corneal surface has been arbitrarily divided into four zones [4] (Fig. 6.1). These divisions are somewhat variable as the corneal surface is smooth, and one zone blends with the next; but the concept is useful when describing the normal corneal shape and has practical applications such as the fitting of contact lenses.

Central Zone

The central zone (otherwise called the apical zone, corneal cap, optical zone, or central spherical zone) is the optically important area about 4 mm diameter which is approximately spherical: its curvature does not vary by more than 0.05 mm (0.25D) [13–15]. This is surrounded by the corneal periphery which is divided into three zones: paracentral, peripheral and limbal.

Paracentral Zone

The paracentral zone is an annulus 4 to 7–8 mm diameter, which normally has a flatter radius of curvature than the central zone. After radial keratotomy, it is the site of the paracentral knee, where there is a marked steepening of the cornea around the flattened central area. Together with the central zone, it forms the apical zone used for contact lens fitting.

Peripheral Zone

The peripheral zone is the area of maximal corneal flattening and radial asymmetry. The peripheral curvature of a contact lens should be fitted to the shape of the cornea in this region, where it obtains most of its support.

Limbal Zone

The limbal zone is a rim 0.5–1 mm wide adjacent to the sclera. It is usually covered by the conjunctival vascular arcade, and its exact extent depends upon the amount of scleral over-ride. Here, there is a focal steepening to form the scleral sulcus. It is a common site for surgical incisions and conditions such as peripheral corneal melts

Topography techniques, such as videokeratoscopy, which are based on the principle of reflection, have difficulty in imaging this area; and even if an image can be obtained, the analysis algorithms are less accurate in the periphery. In contrast, good images can be obtained using projection techniques, and the accuracy of the reconstruction is uniform across the whole area.

The Corneal Centre

The centre of the cornea can be defined in a number of ways. This arises firstly due to the complex shape of the cornea itself, and secondly because the cornea is part of a multicomponent optical system. There are four commonly used corneal centres (Table 6.4), the relative positions of which can vary among individuals [9] (Fig. 6.2).

Table 6.4 Definitions and applications of the corneal centres

Corneal centre		Anterior point	Corneal point	Posterior point	Applications
Geometric corneal centre	GCC		Equidistant from opposite limbuses		Contact lens fitting
Corneal reflex centre	CRC	Fixation point	Corneal apex		Topography
					Hirschberg test (strabismus)
Entrance pupil centre (line of sight)	EPC	Fixation point	Corneal intercept	Entrance pupil centre	Refractive surgery
Visual axis centre	VAC	Fixation point	Corneal intercept	Fovea	Visual function
					Cover test (strabismus)

The axes of the eye are defined by the anterior and posterior points lying on them

Fig. 6.2 Corneal centres. Diagrammatic representation of the right cornea in horizontal section (above) and from anteriorly (below), showing the typical positions of the corneal centres and how they are defined. From inferotemporal to superonasal are the: Geometric Corneal Centre (GCC), Entrance Pupil Centre (EPC), Visual Axis Centre (VAC), and Corneal Reflex Centre (CRC).

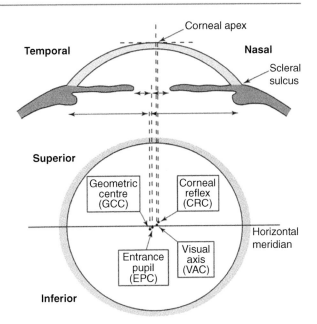

Geometric Corneal Centre

The geometric corneal centre (GCC, or anatomic corneal centre) is where the longest horizontal and vertical surface arcs intersect, or, in other words, the point equidistant from opposite portions of the limbus. It has no special refractive significance as the refractive elements of the eye are not coaxial, but it is used in contact lens fitting.

Corneal Reflex Centre

The coaxially sighted corneal reflex centre (CRC) is, as its name suggests, the site of the corneal light reflex when the cornea is viewed coaxially with the light source. By definition, this is the corneal apex, because when the eye is fixating a light source, the corneal surface will only be perpendicular to approaching light rays at the point of greatest sagittal height [16]. The corneal light reflex is used for centring reflection-based topography systems, such as videokeratoscopes. In conditions like keratoconus, and after refractive surgery, the corneal reflex centre may be markedly displaced from the other corneal centres.

Entrance Pupil Centre

The coaxially sighted entrance pupil centre (EPC) lies at the corneal intercept of a line joining the fixation point with the centre of the pupil. This is called the "line of sight" by some authors, because the pupillary aperture determines the image-forming bundle of rays which reach the retina [17]. However, the ray passing through the centre of the pupil has no special optical significance as to the part of the cornea or retina on which it falls.

The entrance pupil centre is commonly used for centring refractive surgical procedures. This is because the pupil is easy to see, and its use appears to give good clinical results. However, the reliability of this point as a marker of the corneal centre is reduced by its variable position. The centre of the pupil can shift by as much as 0.7 mm with changes in pupillary size, and the direction of the shift can be variable [18].

Visual Axis Centre

The visual axis centre (VAC) lies at the corneal intercept of the visual axis, which connects the fixation point with the fovea. It is assumed to be the centre of the optically important zone of the cornea. If this is true, perhaps refractive surgery procedures should be centred on the visual axis, but this point is difficult to locate clinically. The visual axis centre is most closely approximated by the corneal reflex centre, so some authors suggest that this would be preferable for centring refractive procedures [19–25].

The most common relative positions of the corneal centres are from inferotemporal to superonasal: geometric, entrance pupil, visual axis and corneal reflex [19] (Fig. 6.2). In 21% [26] to 28% [19] of patients, the visual axis and corneal reflex centres are coincident. These metrics significantly affect the performance and outcomes of popular laser-based refractive surgeries in terms of the optical and neural image quality [27, 28].

Identification of Corneal Locations

When describing the topography of a cornea, it is important to be able to unambiguously locate its different features [4].

Meridians

A meridian is a line that spans the diameter of the cornea from one point on the limbus to a point on the opposing limbus. Each is named by the angle it makes with the horizontal, starting with 0° at 3 o'clock, and proceeding to 180°, anticlockwise for both right and left eyes.

A semimeridian lies on a radius, extending from the corneal centre to the limbus, and is labelled from 0 to 360° proceeding anticlockwise from 3 o'clock. Colour-coded contour maps routinely have these positions marked around the periphery of the map (Fig. 6.3).

Axes

An axis is the direction in which a cylindrical lens has no power. When the term is applied to the cornea, it describes the meridian along which the axis of the correcting lens would be placed. For example, if a cornea is steep in the vertical meridian, it would be corrected by a negative cylinder with its axis at 180°.

Polar coordinates are used to describe the position of individual points in terms of their axis and their distance in millimetres from the centre of the cornea. A polar grid consisting of axes and concentric rings 3, 5 and 7 mm in diameter can be

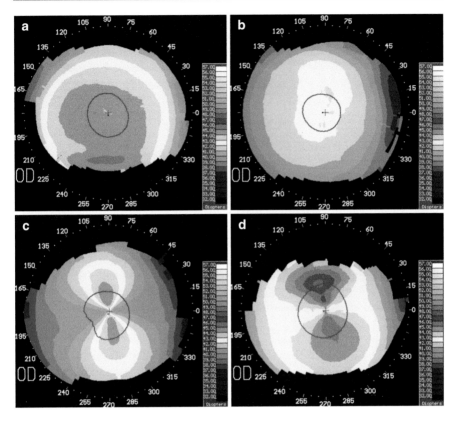

Fig. 6.3 Topography of normal corneas. Normal corneas have been classified as having five types of pattern. (**a**) *Round*. The focal steepening inferiorly is due to the lower tear meniscus. (**b**) *Oval*. (**c**) *Symmetric bow tie*. (**d**) *Asymmetric bow tie*. The bow tie patterns are associated with higher degrees of astigmatism. The fifth pattern is irregular and can have many different appearances. Note the semimeridians labelled in degrees around the periphery of each map

superimposed upon a topography map. The polar coordinates of an individual point can be obtained by marking the point with the cursor and reading the information from the cursor box.

Normal Variations in Corneal Shape

Within a normal population, there are a variety of corneal shapes compatible with good vision. The exact morphology of an individual's corneas is unique [1]. Identification of the extent of the spectrum of normality is necessary before the diagnosis of an abnormal corneal shape can be made. It may also help us to understand the relationship between corneal topography, refractive error and visual function and to determine which topographic characteristics are optically or visually important.

Knoll [29] was the first to propose a classification. From photokeratographs, he categorised patients into four groups on the basis of their central corneal asymmetry and the amount of peripheral flattening along the horizontal meridian. With the advent of the videokeratoscope and more recently, Scheimpflug camera-based devices, it is now possible to make a classification using data from the whole corneal surface.

Classification of Normal Corneas

Bogan and Waring et al. [30] have described five videokeratoscopic patterns which lie on a spectrum of normal corneal shape: round, oval, symmetric bow tie, asymmetric bow tie and irregular (Table 6.5, Fig. 6.3). They examined single eyes of 216 normal individuals. The topography maps were displayed using a normalised scale, in which the scale is automatically adjusted to fill the range of curvatures present on that individual cornea. They classified the cornea according to the shape of the contour corresponding to the middle of the scale. Their classification has since been expanded by other authors [31, 32], and similar methods have been applied to the classification of maps obtained using projection-based techniques [33].

Spherical

In their survey, Bogan et al. found that the predominant pattern was round (Fig. 6.3a) in 22.6%, and oval (Fig. 6.3b) in 20.8%. Surprisingly, patients in these two groups showed no difference in astigmatism, but this may be because both refraction and keratometry make measurements in only a small central area of the cornea.

Table 6.5 Classification and incidence (%) of topographic patterns found in normal corneas, measured by videokeratoscopy [154, 938] and projection techniques [999]

Videokeratoscopy				Projection	
Bogan et al [30]		Rabinowitz et al [31]		Naufal et al [33]	
Spherical					
Round	23	Round	21	Island	29
Oval	21	Oval	25		
		Superior steepening	4		
		Inferior steepening	12		
Astigmatic					
Symmetric bow tie	18	Symmetric bow tie	20	Regular ridge	17
		Symmetric bow tie with skewed axes	2	Incomplete ridge	23
Asymmetric bow tie	32	Asymmetric bow tie, inferior steepening	7	Irregular ridge	28
		Asymmetric bow tie, superior steepening	3		
		Asymmetric bow tie with skewed axes	1		
Irregular					
Irregular	7	Irregular	6	Unclassified	3

Astigmatic

The videokeratoscopy representation of a toric surface has the appearance of a bow tie (Fig. 6.3c, d), with the bows of the tie aligned along the steeper meridian (Chap. 1). This configuration arises from the fact that videokeratoscopes use a reflected image to measure the slope of a surface and express the result as radius of curvature. In contrast, projection-based systems, which measure the corneal height, depict a toric surface as a series of concentric ellipses with their long axis in the flatter meridian, similar to the contours of a geographical ordinance survey map. If a best-fit sphere is subtracted from the corneal height data, astigmatism appears as a ridge [33].

In Bogan's study [30], a bow tie pattern was present in 49.6% of patients (symmetric bow tie in 17.5%, asymmetric bow tie in 32.1%). Astigmatism was much more common in this group, particularly in those with symmetric bow ties (Fig. 6.3c). In patients with bow tie patterns but no astigmatism, one must assume that either the central portion of the cornea is spherical or that the corneal toricity is matched by inverse lenticular astigmatism (the incidence of keratometric astigmatism was higher than for refractive astigmatism).

In a normal eye, an asymmetric bow tie (Fig. 6.3d) represents radial asymmetry in the rate of change of the radius of curvature from centre to periphery. The same pattern is also obtained in cases of contact lens warpage or early keratoconus, or as an artefact due to eccentric fixation by the subject or decentration by the operator. This demonstrates how the boundaries between normality and disease are not always easily defined and that a diagnosis should not be made on the topography alone, but in conjunction with the clinical history and examination.

7.1% of patients had an irregular pattern which did not match any of the other four patterns. Surface irregularity can also result from eccentric fixation, improper focusing or tear film abnormalities.

Enantiomorphism

Bogan found a striking degree of similarity between the two eyes of the same individual (Fig. 6.4). In 60% of subjects, both eyes were assigned to the same group, and in 79%, both eyes were either round/oval or bow tie or irregular. An individual's corneas are frequently enantiomorphic: the topography of one cornea is the mirror image of the fellow eye [1]. This is not surprising when one considers that other anatomical structures such as ears or fingerprints also display enantiomorphism. It can be helpful to utilise this feature when deciding whether a cornea is normal or not, by comparing its topography with that of the fellow eye.

Variations in the Shape of Individual Corneas

Lifetime Variation

Small changes in corneal astigmatism occur throughout life. In infancy, the cornea is fairly spherical. During childhood and adolescence, it becomes astigmatic "with-the-rule": in about 90% of individuals, the cornea is steepest in the vertical

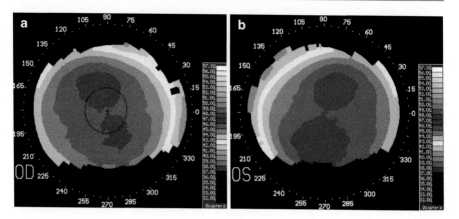

Fig. 6.4 Enantiomorphism. The right (**a**) and left (**b**) eyes of the same individual commonly show mirror image topography. This patient's spectacle prescription included a −2.00D cylinder at axis 20° for the right eye and160° for the left eye. In cases of corneal disease or surgery, it is useful to compare the topography of the eye being studied with the normal other eye. This gives an idea of how the topography of the affected eye might have been previously

meridian, which is corrected by a negative cylinder at axis 180°. This may possibly result from eyelid pressure. Sphericity tends to return during middle age, and astigmatism "against-the-rule" may develop later in life [34, 35].

Short-Term Fluctuations
Natural short-term fluctuations in corneal morphology are usually unnoticed by individuals with normal corneas but may become apparent in conditions such as bullous keratopathy, Fuchs' endothelial dystrophy or contact lens intolerance.

Diurnal Variation
Diurnal variations in corneal curvature and thickness are thought to be caused by the period of lid closure during sleep. Overnight, reduced tear evaporation and possibly changes in tear tonicity lead to a thickening of both central and peripheral cornea by about 3–8%. This usually returns towards normal within about 2 h of lid opening and then remains fairly stable for the rest of the day. Lid pressure may cause a flattening of the central cornea during sleep, which then slowly reverses throughout the day, although no change in surface asphericity has been detected [36, 37]. It has been suggested that lifting the eyelid away from the cornea might cause corneal steepening [38], but no correlation has been found between eyelid tension and corneal toricity [12].

Menstrual Variation

The presence and extent of corneal changes detected during the menstrual cycle varies between authors [39–42]. Some have correlated serum oestrogen levels with flattening and an increased thickness of the cornea. This could be explained by oestrogens increasing the hydration of the cornea, as they do in other tissues. These changes, if real, are so small that they are almost beyond the limit of detection of topography systems and are unlikely to be of clinical significance in normal eyes.

Contact Lens-Induced Corneal Warpage

Of much greater importance than the natural variations in corneal shape are those that arise as a result of both PMMA and hydrogel contact lens wear (Chap. 7) [43]. Corneal warpage probably occurs as a direct result of mechanical pressure from the contact lens, but metabolic factors, such as low oxygen tension, have not been excluded. Patients are commonly asymptomatic [44], but some lose as many as four Snellen lines of best spectacle-corrected visual acuity or develop contact lens intolerance [45].

Artefacts of Corneal Topography

The previous section described the range of topographic appearances of a normal cornea. However, a pattern outside this spectrum does not necessarily imply that the cornea is abnormal. It is important to be able to recognise when topographic irregularities are due to external influences, rather than the cornea itself.

Alignment and Focusing

The acquisition of accurate topography is dependent upon the care of the operator and the cooperation of the patient. In videokeratoscopy and Scheimpflug-based systems, the cornea must be correctly positioned relative to the cone to fulfil many of the assumptions made by the reconstruction algorithms (Chaps. 2 and 4). The patient must maintain fixation of the target, and the equipment must be properly centred and focused. Small errors in alignment can result in an irregular or asymmetric topographic reconstruction [46–49] (Fig. 6.5). In addition, blinking or eye movement can lead to data gaps and a poor quality scan.

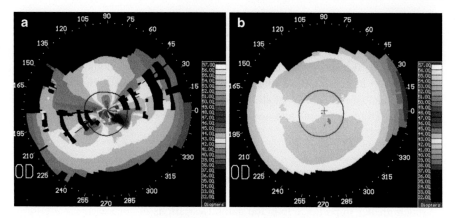

Fig. 6.5 Misalignment. (**a**) When the patient fixates eccentrically or the Placido cone is misaligned relative to the cornea, the topography cannot be accurately reconstructed. (**b**) When these errors were corrected, the patient was shown to have a normal regular cornea

Fig. 6.6 Tear film drying. Localised drying of the tear film causes focal areas of flattening. These commonly occur over the steepest or most prominent parts of the cornea. If drying causes excessive irregularity, reconstruction may be inaccurate or impossible in that area

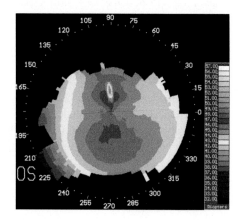

Tear Film Irregularities

Another cause of spurious topography is irregularities of the tear film, because videokeratoscopes image the air-tear fluid interface rather than the corneal epithelium [50–52]. Pooling of tears in the lower meniscus produces a focal steepening (Fig. 6.3a), and thinning of the tear film by drying shows as a localised flattening of the surface (Fig. 6.6). Poor tear quality can interfere with the accuracy of the measurements in a less specific manner (Fig. 6.7a, b). These artefacts can be overcome by asking the patient to blink immediately before the image is captured (Fig. 6.7c).

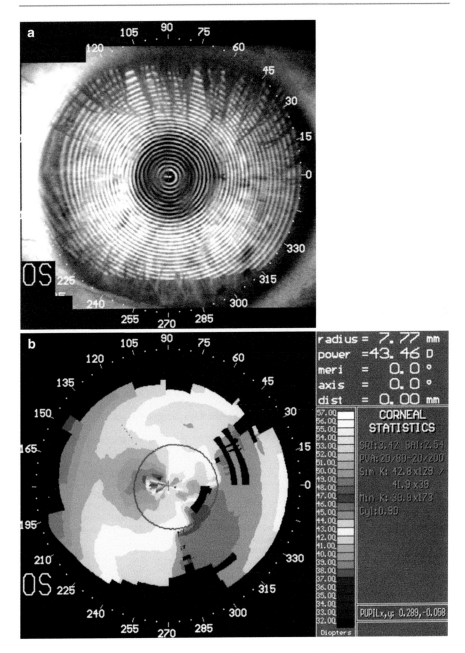

Fig. 6.7 Tear film irregularity. At an examination after photorefractive keratectomy, the first colour map (**b**) showed marked surface irregularity, as supported by the statistical indices. Reversion to the videokeratograph (**a**) revealed dark oily swirls in the tear film. The patient was asked to blink several times, and then the repeat colour map (**c**) confirmed a regular corneal surface

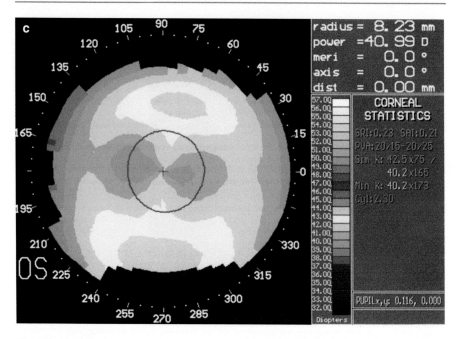

Fig. 6.7 (continued)

References
References Particularly Worth Reading

1. *Dingeldein SA, Klyce SD. The topography of normal corneas. Arch Ophthalmol 1989; 107: 512–518.
2. Fleming JF. Should refractive surgeons worry about corneal asphericity? Refract Corneal Surg. 1990;6:455–7.
3. Carney LG, Mainstone JC, Henderson BA. Corneal topography and myopia: a cross-sectional study. Invest Ophthalmol Vis Sci. 1997;38:311–20.
4. *Waring GO. Making sense of keratospeak II: proposed conventional terminology for corneal topography. Refract Corneal Surg 1989; 5: 362–367.
5. Eghbali F, Yeung KK, Maloney RK. Topographic determination of corneal asphericity and its lack of effect on the outcome of radial keratotomy. Am J Ophthalmol. 1995;119:275–80.
6. Edmund C, Sjontoft E. The central-peripheral radius of the normal corneal curvature: a photo-keratoscopic study. Acta Ophthalmol. 1985;63:670–7.
7. Wang J, Rice DA, Klyce SD. A new reconstruction algorithm for improvement of corneal topographical analysis. Refract Corneal Surg. 1989;5:379–87.
8. Holladay JT. Corneal topography using the Holladay diagnostic summary. J Cat Refract Surg. 1997;23:209–21.
9. Duke-Elder S. System of ophthalmology. Vol V: ophthalmic optics and refraction. St Louis: CV Mosby; 1970. p. 274–95.
10. Young T. The mechanisms of the eye. Philos Trans. 1801;91:23.
11. Donders F. On the anomalies of refraction and accommodation of the eye. London: The New Sydenham Society; 1864.

12. Fredrick S, Wilson G. The relation between eyelid tension, corneal toricity, and age. Invest Ophthalmol Vis Sci. 1983;24:1367–73.
13. Mandell RB, St Helen R. Stability of the corneal contour. Am J Optom. 1968;45:797–806.
14. Clark BA. Mean topography of normal corneas. Aust J Optom. 1974;57:107–14.
15. Clark BA. Topography of some individual corneas. Aust J Optom. 1974;57:65–9.
16. Mandell RB, St Helen R. Position and curvature of the corneal apex. Am J Optom. 1969;46:25–7.
17. *Uozato H, Guyton DL. Centring corneal surgical procedures. Am J Ophthalmol 1987; 103: 264–275.
18. Fay AM, Trokel SL, Myers JA. Pupil diameter and the principal ray. J Cat Refract Surg. 1992;18:348–51.
19. *Pande M, Hillman JS. Optical zone centration in keratorefractive surgery. Ophthalmology 1993; 100: 1230–1237.
20. Doane JF, Cavanaugh TB. Optical zone centration for keratorefractive surgery [letter]. Ophthalmology. 1994;101:215–6.
21. Pande M. Optical zone centration for keratorefractive surgery [reply]. Ophthalmology. 1994;101:216.
22. Mandell RB. Optical zone centration for keratorefractive surgery [letter]. Ophthalmology. 1994;101:216–7.
23. Pande M. Optical zone centration for keratorefractive surgery [reply]. Ophthalmology. 1994;101:217–9.
24. Guyton DL. More on optical zone centration [letter]. Ophthalmology. 1994;101:793.
25. Pande M, Hillman JS. More on optical zone centration [reply]. Ophthalmology. 1994;101:793–4.
26. Tomlinson A, Schwartz C. The position of the corneal apex in the normal eye. Am J Optom Phys Optics. 1979;56:236–40.
27. McAlinden C. Corneal refractive surgery: past to present. Clin Exp Optom. 2012;95(4):386–98.
28. Mosquera SA, Verma S, McAlinden C. Centration axis in refractive surgery. Eye Vis (Lond). 2015;2:4.
29. Knoll HA. Corneal contours in the general population as revealed by the photokeratoscope. Am J Optom. 1961;38:389–97.
30. *Bogan SJ, Waring GO, Ibrahim O, Drews C, Curtis L. Classification of normal corneal topography based on computer-assisted videokeratography. Arch Ophthalmol 1990; 108: 945–949.
31. Rabinowitz YS, Yang H, Brickman Y, Akkina J, Riley C, Rotter JI, Elashoff J. Videokeratography database of normal human corneas. Br J Ophthalmol. 1996;80:610–6.
32. Alvi NP, McMahon TT, Devulappally J, Chen TC, Vianna MAG. Characteristics of normal corneal topography using the EyeSys corneal analysis system. J Cataract Refract Surg. 1997;23:849–55.
33. *Naufal SC, Hess JS, Friedlander MH, Granet NS. Rasterstereography-based classification of normal corneas. J Cataract Refract Surg 1997; 23: 222–230.
34. Marin-Amat M. The physiological variations of the corneal curvature during life, their significance in ocular refraction. Bull Soc Belg Ophthalmol. 1957;136:263.
35. Sawada A. Refractive errors in an elderly Japanese population: the Tajimi study. Ophthalmology. 2008;115(2):363–70.
36. Kiely PM, Carney LG, Smith G. Diurnal variations of corneal topography and thickness. Am J Optom Physiol Optic. 1982;59:976–82.
37. Read SA, Collins MJ, Carney LG. The diurnal variation of corneal topography and aberrations. Cornea. 2005;24(6):678–87.
38. Clark BAJ. Variations in corneal topography. Aust J Optom. 1973;56:399–413.
39. El Hage SD, Beaulne C. Changes in central and peripheral corneal thickness with menstrual cycle. Am J Optom Physiol Optic. 1973;50:863–71.
40. Kiely PM, Carney LG, Smith G. Menstrual cycle variations of corneal topography and thickness. Am J Optom Physiol Optic. 1983;60:822–9.
41. Giuffrè G, Di Rosa L, Fiorino F, Bubella DM, Lodato G. Variations in central corneal thickness during the menstrual cycle in women. Cornea. 2007;26(2):144–6.

42. Ghahfarokhi NA, Vaseghi A, Ghoreishi M, et al. Evaluation of corneal thickness alterations during menstrual cycle in productive age women. Indian J Ophthalmol. 2015;63(1):30–2.
43. Schornack M. Hydrogel contact lens-induced corneal warpage. Cont Lens Anterior Eye. 2003;26(3):153–9.
44. Ruiz-Montenegro J, Mafra CH, Wilson SE, Jumper JM, Klyce SD, Mendelson EN. Corneal topographic alterations in normal contact lens wearers. Ophthalmology. 1993;100:128–34.
45. Wilson SE, Lin DTC, Klyce SD, Reidy JJ, Insler MS. Topographic changes in contact lens-induced warpage. Ophthalmology. 1990;97:734–44.
46. Wang J, Rice DA, Klyce SD. Analysis of the effects of astigmatism and misalignment on corneal surface reconstruction from photokeratoscopic data. Refract Corneal Surg. 1991;7:129–40.
47. *Hubbe RE, Foulks GN. The effect of poor fixation on computer-assisted topographic corneal analysis. Ophthalmology 1994; 101: 1745–1748.
48. Singh D. Effect of cataract on corneal topography results. J Cataract Refract Surg. 1996;22:1506–8.
49. Karabatsas CH, Hoh HB. Is it cataract or misalignment that affects corneal topography measurements? [letter]. J Cataract Refract Surg. 1997;23:694–5.
50. Mishima S. Some physiological aspects of the precorneal tearfilm. Arch Ophthalmol. 1965;73:233.
51. *Pavlopoulos GP, Horn J, Feldman ST. The effect of artificial tears on computer-assisted corneal topography in normal eyes and after penetrating keratoplasty. Am J Ophthalmol 1995; 119: 712–722.
52. Novak KD, Kohnen T, Chang-Godinich A, Soper BA, Kennedy P, Wang Q, Padrick T, Koch DD. Changes in computerised videokeratography induced by artificial tears. J Cat Refract Surg. 1997;23:1023–8.

Contact Lens Practice

7

Corneal topography can have a role in both the fitting of contact lenses and the monitoring of the corneal profile thereafter. Many topography systems have contact lens fitting programmes incorporated into their software to facilitate these options.

When corneal contact lenses were first introduced in the 1950s, measurements of the anterior surface of the cornea and the posterior surface of the contact lenses were expressed in terms of radius of curvature. This method is still largely used today, although newer topography systems which assess true corneal shape in terms of height are useful for the more complex corneal shapes occurring as a result of disease or surgery (Chap. 5).

Contact Lens Types

Early contact lenses were made of polymethylmethacrylate (PMMA). Although this material is still available, it is no longer considered suitable for contact lenses, due to its lack of oxygen permeability (Table 7.1). The development of rigid materials with higher oxygen permeabilities leads to the introduction of rigid gas permeable (RGP) lenses, which give a greater range of fitting options to the practitioner. These remain useful for the correction of regular and irregular astigmatism and in complicated cases requiring scleral lenses.

Contact lens practice has changed dramatically since the advent of the soft lens in the early 1970s. Whilst rigid gas permeable (RGP) lenses are relatively popular in Europe, soft lenses have obtained up to an 80% share of the market in some countries [1]. Two main reasons for the popularity of soft lenses have been their initial comfort and their ease of fitting. Soft lens use has also been enhanced by the advent of daily disposable lenses and multipurpose care solutions, but they are only useful for regular corneas. Typically, disposable soft lenses are 'one-fit' lenses with few lens design options available, and therefore fitting does not require topographic measurements.

© Springer Nature Switzerland AG 2019
M. Corbett et al., *Corneal Topography*,
https://doi.org/10.1007/978-3-030-10696-6_7

Table 7.1 Comparison of different types of contact lenses

Contact lens type	Advantages	Disadvantages
Hard (PMMA)	Good visual performance	Low oxygen permeability
		Limited fitting options
		Contact lens-induced warpage
Rigid gas permeable (RGP)	Good visual performance	Individualised fitting required
	Higher oxygen permeability than hard	Contact lens-induced warpage
	Custom lens designs possible	
	Lenses can be modified/polished	
	Good lens solution compatibility	
Soft	Good oxygen permeability	More ocular infections
	Good tolerance	
	Easy to fit	
	Good for use in sport	

PMMA polymethylmethacrylate

However, there has been concern about the relatively high incidence of ocular infections, including microbial keratitis, associated with soft contact lens wear [2–7]. It is evident from both published studies and clinical experience that RGP lenses are much less likely to be associated with this problem and therefore provide a safer option. As RGP lenses have some significant clinical advantages over soft lenses, it has been important to further simplify their fitting so that this may be performed by relatively inexperienced practitioners.

Contact Lens Designs

When fitting RGP lenses, the posterior surface (lens base curve) should be shaped appropriately for the cornea, and then the power selected (back vertex power, BVP) is determined by the curvature of the anterior surface (Fig. 7.1). This can be measured by keratometry in normal corneas, but it is preferable to use topography in irregular corneas.

In recent years, there have been two developments which have facilitated the fitting of RGP lenses. Firstly, corneal topography can provide detailed information about the configuration of the anterior corneal surface. Secondly, RGP lenses have become available with a series of standard back surface designs which are intended to fit the majority of normal corneas, or a particular group of abnormal corneas, such as keratoconus, post-graft, or reverse geometry lenses for very flat corneas including those after refractive surgery. Keratometry may be sufficient for fitting RGP lenses in regular corneas, but topography is preferable for fitting irregular corneas.

Fig. 7.1 Contact lens structure. Cross section through a rigid gas permeable lens of positive power. (**a**) It has a tricurve back surface where the more peripheral curves are flatter to give a degree of edge lift. The front surface has two zones of different curvature. (**b**) When prescribing contact lenses, the dimensions required also need to be stated

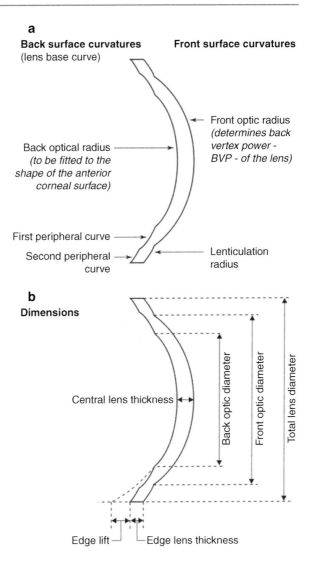

a

Back surface curvatures (lens base curve)

Front surface curvatures

Front optic radius (determines back vertex power - BVP - of the lens)

Back optical radius (to be fitted to the shape of the anterior corneal surface)

First peripheral curve

Second peripheral curve

Lenticulation radius

b

Dimensions

Central lens thickness

Back optic diameter

Front optic diameter

Total lens diameter

Edge lift

Edge lens thickness

Anterior Surface

The front curve of a contact lens is lenticulated and governs its back vertex power (BVP). In positive lenses, the front optic radius is steeper than the back optic radius, so the lens is thicker in the centre than the periphery (Fig. 7.1). The reverse is true of negative lenses. Outside the front optic diameter is a portion of no optical importance which is referred to as the lenticular carrier.

Posterior Surface

The base curve of a contact lens determines the shape of its posterior surface. This is commonly composed of two or more curves of different radii so that it can be fitted to the cornea to provide edge clearance. The central zone of the lens, with a curvature determined by the back optic radius, is the zone of optical importance. The peripheral zones have increasingly flatter radii of curvature to accommodate the prolate shape of the cornea. The edge lift is an axial measure of the distance by which the edge of the lens back surface deviates from a sphere. These can be varied independently of the back optic radius.

The relationship of the lens base curve to the cornea becomes particularly complicated when fitting special designs, such as toric or bifocal lenses. However, new lathing technology has now enabled lens back surfaces to be accurately generated with aspheric curves or with a combination of a spheric optic and an aspheric periphery.

Early lens designs were created for PMMA lenses in the 1960s and 1970 [8]. The concept of constant axial edge lift lenses was developed and has remained largely unaltered in current RGP lens designs. Only two significant changes have been made. Firstly, there has been a reduction in the degree of edge lift to aid comfort. Secondly, the higher oxygen permeability of the material has enabled the back optic zone diameter to be increased to give better pupil coverage or the overall diameter to be increased to improve lens stability over irregular corneas. Hybrid lenses with a rigid centre and soft peripheral skirt aim to combine good vision with improved fit and comfort. However, even the more modern versions are still associated with relatively high complication rates, such as corneal vascularisation due to reduced oxygen permeability.

Tear Layer Thickness

A contact lens is only in contact with the cornea over a small portion of its posterior surface. Over the remaining area, the space in between the lens and the cornea is filled by tear fluid (Fig. 7.2). An RGP contact lens can correct astigmatism because its anterior surface is usually spherical, and the trapped tear layer fills any irregularities between the posterior lens surface and the anterior cornea. The interface with the greatest change in refractive index, and therefore the greatest optical power, is that between the air and the anterior surface of the contact lens, which is spherical. The lens, tear film and cornea are of similar refractive index and therefore act as a single optical component with a spherical front surface.

Custom Design Lenses

If a toric back surface has to be used to give a better physical fit in a case of corneal astigmatism (>3D), then the anterior surface of the tear layer will be toric, and induced astigmatism may result. This can be corrected by the front of the lens being cylindrical [9].

With the increasing sophistication of corneal topography systems, it should be possible for their software to design the appropriate RGP lens for an individual cornea

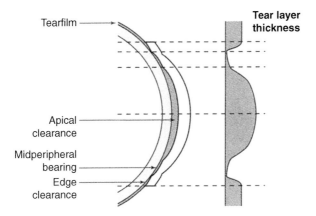

Fig. 7.2 Tear layer thickness. Cross section through a hard contact lens fitted with minimal apical clearance, midperipheral bearing and a degree of edge clearance (left). Tear fluid fills in the space between the contact lens and the cornea. The thickness of this layer (right) determines the fluorescein pattern: the areas with a thick tear layer appear green, whereas the areas of bearing appear black

and to control the lathing machine to produce a tailor-made lens. Videokeratoscopes based on Placido disc technology may not be sufficiently accurate in their reconstructions, particularly in the periphery of the aspheric cornea, to be used for this purpose (Chap. 2). However, the development of Scheimpflug and projection-based systems which measure the true corneal shape in terms of height may show more promise in this field (Chap. 3).

Contact Lens Fitting

For the eye care practitioner involved in contact lens practice, the most likely clinical uses of corneal topography are in relation to the fitting of RGP lenses and in the follow-up and aftercare procedures of all types of contact lenses. However, in routine contact lens cases, keratometry remains the most common method for assessing corneal curvature.

Assessment of Fit

Contact lens fitting involves a series of steps, each of which is usually followed by a trial of a contact lens in the eye (Fig. 7.3). Corneal topography makes this process more efficient by using detailed measurements and computer simulations of the fluorescein fitting patterns, thereby reducing the number of lens trials necessary. This is more comfortable for the patient and, by minimising the time spent on routine cases, leaves the practitioner more time for the difficult cases that require

Fig. 7.3 Contact lens fitting process. The greater detail provided by corneal topography compared to keratometry reduces the number of trial lenses required to obtain a good fit

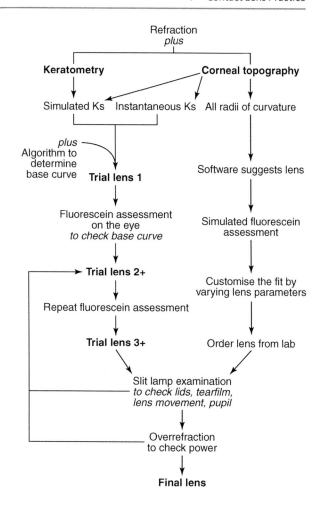

greater individual attention. Although topography is a useful tool which can assist the clinician, it is unlikely to replace the experienced contact lens fitter.

Corneal Curvature

At present keratometry is routinely used by contact lens practitioners to measure central corneal curvature and provide a starting point in choosing a rigid lens fitting. However, the 'K' readings assume a spherical or spherocylindrical surface and measure corneal curvature at only four points, 3 mm apart in the paracentral cornea (Chap. 2). The information would be adequate if all corneas had spherical or spherocylindrical surfaces. However the cornea is aspheric and radially asymmetric, conforming most closely to a flattening ellipse (Chap. 6). Therefore, more information, particularly about the corneal periphery, can be provided by topography. This is useful in irregular corneas, such as keratoconus, in which the curvature of the steepest part of the cone can be identified.

Fitting Nomograms

'K readings' from a keratometer, or simulated Ks from topography, can be entered into an algorithm which determines the base curve most likely to fit the cornea. However, if topography is used, the software automatically suggests the most appropriate lens. This can be further refined by entering other variables such as the refraction and the pupil diameter. Some programmes suggest alternative lenses, such as the one giving the best central fit, based upon an individual lens design.

Simulated Fluorescein Patterns

The application of fluorescein to the tear film shows the thickness of the tear layer and therefore the proximity of the posterior surface of the lens to the anterior surface of the cornea (Fig. 7.2). Where the tear layer is thicker, it appears bright green, and where it is thinner or in areas of lenticulo-corneal touch, it appears darker. The screen display of the simulated fluorescein pattern enables this information to be obtained without inserting a trial lens (Figs. 7.4, 7.5 and 7.6). This may help avoid excessive trials and determine the best static lens fit, particularly in difficult cases where there is unusual corneal topography, such as in keratoconus or following keratoplasty. The simulated fluorescein patterns can also be based on the chosen fitting philosophy of the individual practitioner, such as an alignment fit or apical clearance fit.

Different back surface curvatures can be entered to demonstrate the fluorescein pattern produced by various lenses. These can be displayed in conjunction with the measured topography, so the back surface curvature can be titrated against the fluorescein pattern. In some systems, aspherical as well as spherical back surfaces can be selected.

Lens Dynamics

Some software has now introduced pan-and-tilt features in an attempt to replicate the actual position of the lens on the cornea. This gives a more realistic impression of the true dynamic fit of the lens [10].

Slit-Lamp Examination

Currently the effect of other variables such as lens movement, tear dynamics and lid configuration (position and tension) have to be observed on biomicroscopic slit-lamp examination [11]. However, as more information is collected by these systems, it is likely that the software will be further developed to include these variables.

Over-refraction

Once the posterior surface of the contact lens has been fitted to the cornea, it is necessary to confirm that the lens is of the appropriate power. The refractive effect of a contact lens in situ is a combination of the power of the lens itself and the power of the tear layer trapped beneath it:

Corrected Refractive Error = Contact Lens Power + Liquid Lens Power

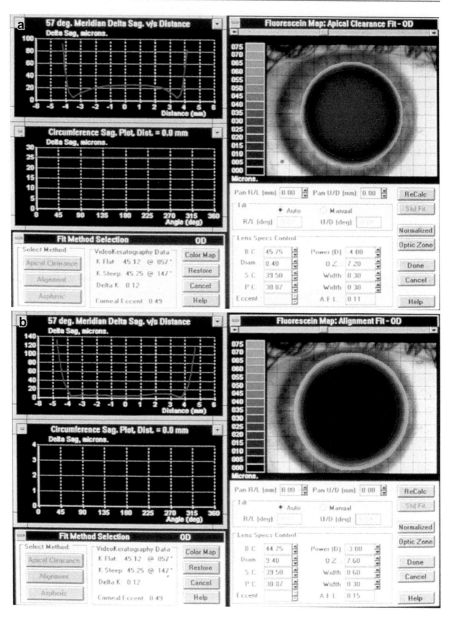

Fig. 7.4 Simulated fluorescein pattern. Simulated fluorescein fit of a rigid gas permeable contact lens on a normal cornea. The topographic simulated keratometry data are displayed (bottom left), and the lens parameters can be altered (bottom right). The associated fluorescein map is shown (top right), together with a graph of the tear layer thickness across the centre of the lens (top left) or circumferentially at a given zone (middle left). (**a**) In an apical clearance fit, tear fluid collects under the centre of the lens, which therefore appears green. The peripheral area of marginal bearing remains dark. (**b**) In an apical bearing (alignment) fit, the centre of the contact lens is close to the corneal apex, and this therefore appears dark due to the tear layer being thin

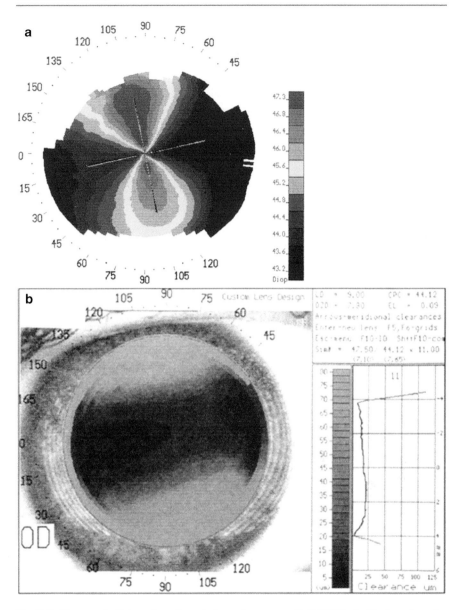

Fig. 7.5 Fluorescein fit in astigmatism. Astigmatic cornea with 3.50DC of with-the-rule astigmatism. (**a**) Colour-coded power map with orgonal axes indicating the major and minor meridia. (Corneal statistics: SRI = 0.56, SAI = 0.21; PVA 20/20–20/25; SimK = 47.2×11°; MinK = 43.8×4°). (**b**) Simulated fluorescein pattern of a spherical RGP lens fitted with a base curve aligning the flat meridian of the cornea. The tear layer is thinnest in a horizontal band, and there is excessive edge clearance in the steep meridian. (**c**) Simulated fluorescein pattern with a lens chosen to fit the mean K. This demonstrates the uneven bearing area and the variation in edge clearance

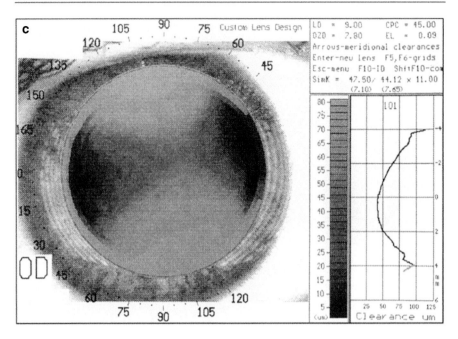

Fig. 7.5 (continued)

Although the patients' spectacle correction is input to the software, the appropriate correction of the refractive error can be confirmed by performing an over-refraction with the contact lens in situ.

Clinical Effectiveness

The clinical effectiveness of contact fitting can be assessed in several ways. Commonly it is expressed as the proportion of patients in whom the first fit is correct. Alternative measures include the number of changes to lens parameters which have to be made before the correct fit is established or the time taken.

Using keratometry and a nomogram, the success rate of the first fit is 25–60% [12–14]. This compares to 90–95% when the remaining steps of the fitting procedure are complete. Videokeratoscopy produces a successful first fit in 77% of patients with normal corneas [13, 15]. There was also a 50% reduction in 'chair time' relative to traditional methods of fitting. The main advantage of using topography for fitting is that a patient can try lenses which should fit rather than lenses from a trial set which are likely to be at best an approximation of fit and back vertex power. Ideally the same trial needs to be performed on irregular corneas, following corneal disease or surgery.

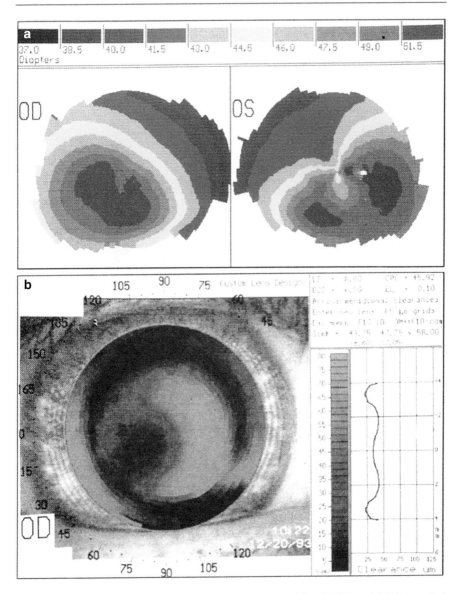

Fig. 7.6 Fluorescein fit in keratoconus. Bilateral keratoconus with an RGP lens. (**a**) Colour-coded maps show significant inferior corneal steepening bilaterally. (**b**) An apical bearing fit of an RGP spherical lens in right eye shows central touch. This is confirmed by there being very little clearance on the tear layer thickness graph to the right. (**c**) An apical clearance fit in the same eye requires a very steep contact lens. This gives a tight fit, particularly in the midperiphery and at the edge of the lens, where little fluorescein is evident

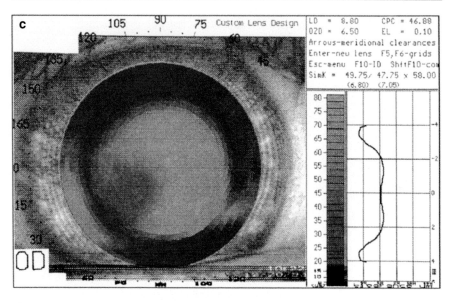

Fig. 76 (continued)

The lower success rate of topographic fitting alone compared to full clinical fitting is due to the absence of parameters in the software relating to lens dynamics or lid configuration. However, this is easily rectified by observing the dynamics of the recommended lens on the eye and performing an over-refraction. Such a combined approach allows the minimum number of trial lenses to be used before the final lens specifications are determined.

Fitting Philosophies

The posterior surface of a contact lens does not exactly fit the anterior surface of the cornea, and therefore the two are closer together in some areas than others. The areas of bearing, where the two are closest, vary with their relative curvatures. The back surface curvature of the contact lens can be selected by the practitioner to give the required characteristics.

Apical Clearance Fit

A lens which is steeper than the corneal apex results in apical clearance (i.e. tear pooling and therefore maximum fluorescein staining at the apex) and marginal bearing (i.e. dark periphery on the fluorescein simulation) (Fig. 7.4a). Such a lens tends to centre well, but tear exchange may be limited [16].

Apical Bearing Fit

A flatter lens gives an apical bearing fit, in which the centre of the lens is aligned with the cornea. The tear layer is thinnest in the area of apical bearing (dark centrally on simulated fluorescein) (Fig. 7.4b). Better tear exchange occurs as a result of greater mobility of the lens and thicker tear layer in the periphery (marginal fluorescence).

Fitting Astigmatic Corneas

Corneal topography determines that portion of the total ocular astigmatism, as measured by refraction, which is due to astigmatism of the cornea. This helps select the most appropriate contact lens type (hard or soft, spherical or toric) for the shape of the cornea and to correct the astigmatism.

The most common type of ocular astigmatism is with-the-rule (steep in the vertical meridian), and this is usually largely due to corneal astigmatism (Chap. 6). In contrast, against-the-rule astigmatism (flat in the vertical meridian) is commonly partly corneal and partly lenticular in origin. In these cases, if the corneal astigmatism was neutralised by a contact lens, residual astigmatism would still persist.

If a lens with a spherical back surface is selected, the base curve may be fitted either to the flat meridian or to the mean keratometry reading. A base curve fitting the flat meridian leaves excess edge clearance on the steep meridian (Fig. 7.5b). However, a base curve equivalent to the mean keratometry reading produces increased bearing in the flat meridian (Fig. 7.5c). It is evident that in an eye with a moderate degree of corneal astigmatism, a spherical lens is a compromise. The only means of achieving an even bearing surface across the back surface of the lens, and therefore a better physical fit, would be to use a toric lens to match the toricity of the eye. This will be facilitated by the availability of toric lens fitting options on video-keratoscopic fluorescein simulation software.

Fitting Keratoconus

Keratoconic corneas show greater than normal variation in curvature from the centre to the periphery and generally have irregular astigmatism (Chap. 10). Contact lenses are usually fitted with a mild apical bearing pattern. In this situation, the fluorescein simulation shows light central touch and a marginal rim of fluorescence (Fig. 7.6b). A steeper lens may be fitted with the aim of giving apical clearance and better centration. However, this causes a large area of lens-corneal contact in the periphery (Fig. 7.6c), giving rise to poor lens mobility, reduced tear exchange and often less good vision.

In order to facilitate the fitting of complex corneas such as these, some video-keratoscopic software has increased the number of curves on the back surface which can be selected. In keratoconus it is useful to try small back optic zones and to move the lens around to assess the fit. It is possible to custom-design lenses to suit the topography.

Fitting Irregular Corneas

The pan-and-tilt features of some of the new software can be used to assess the dynamic fit of the lens and demonstrate how the fluorescein pattern varies with different lens positions (Fig. 7.7).

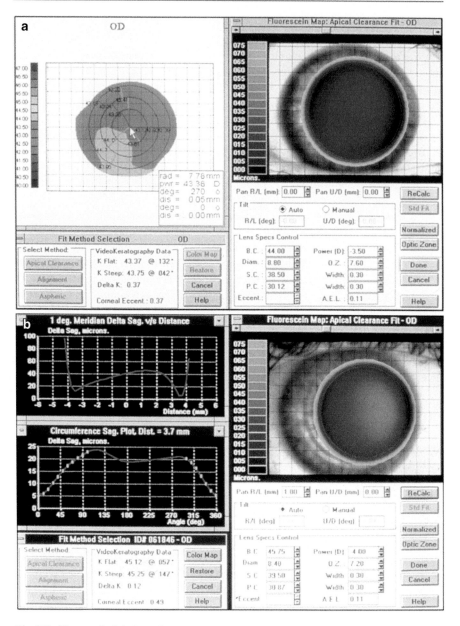

Fig. 7.7 Fluorescein fit in irregular corneas. Mild irregular astigmatism with an RGP lens. (**a**) The colour map can be viewed alongside the fluorescein simulation. (**b**) The "pan" function (box immediately beneath the fluorescein simulation) has been used to displace the lens nasally by 1 mm. There is now greater bearing on the temporal than the nasal side

Contact Lens Front Surface Topography

The shape of the front surface of a contact lens can be assessed by measuring topography with the contact lens in situ. This assesses the air-tear film interface on the surface of the lens, rather than the air-tear film interface on the cornea. This can be helpful when evaluating lens flexure or in correlating lens front surface astigmatism with the uncorrected ocular astigmatism found on over-refraction.

The front surface of toric soft lenses can be tested on the eye to assess if astigmatism has been neutralised by a particular lens design [17]. This function may be more relevant to lens designers and manufacturers rather than clinicians.

Monitoring Corneal Topography

Although the specialist contact lens software in corneal topography systems relates to the fitting of RGP lenses, the standard colour-coded topography maps can be valuable in the follow-up and aftercare of patients wearing all kinds of lenses. Monitoring corneal topography in contact lens wear is helpful in the refractive management of a patient.

Contact Lens-Induced Corneal Warpage

Contact lens wear can alter the shape of the cornea by a process termed warpage [18]. This is thought to occur as a direct result of mechanical pressure from the lens, but metabolic factors, such as low oxygen tension, have not been excluded. Patients are commonly asymptomatic [19], but some lose as many as four Snellen lines of best spectacle-corrected visual acuity or develop contact lens intolerance [20]. In a patient who complains of deteriorating vision with spectacles, whilst maintaining good contact lens acuity, corneal warpage should be suspected.

Topographic abnormalities are most common, severe and persistent in wearers of hard or rigid gas permeable lenses. Many topographic patterns can result, but they tend to comprise flattening in the areas of lens-bearing, with possible adjacent steepening (Table 7.2, Fig. 7.8). For example, a superior-riding contact lens may

Table 7.2 Topographic patterns induced by contact lens wear as a result of corneal warpage

Patterns of contact lens-induced corneal warpage
Central irregular astigmatism
Change in the axis of astigmatism
Radial asymmetry
Reversal of the normal pattern of progressive flattening from the centre to the periphery (i.e. oblate rather than prolate)
Relative flattening beneath the most frequent resting position of the contact lens, especially if it is decentred
Relative steepening outside the resting position of the lens

Fig. 7.8 Contact lens-induced corneal warpage. Wearers of PMMA or RGP lenses can develop a variety of changes in their corneal topography, depending on the fit and position of their lens. (**a**) Inferior flattening in a patient who had been wearing RGP lenses for 1 h since the topography in Fig. 6.4 was taken. (**b**) Superior flattening and inferior steepening causing radial asymmetry as a result of a superior-riding contact lens. This appearance could be confused with that of keratoconus. The patient had been wearing contact lenses for 21 years and had a similar appearance in the other eye. The surface regularity and asymmetry indices were elevated, and the predicted visual acuity was 20/30–20/40. (**c**) Central corneal flattening giving rise to irregular astigmatism with a broken bow tie appearance. The cornea is oblate (flatter in the centre than the periphery) rather than prolate like normal corneas

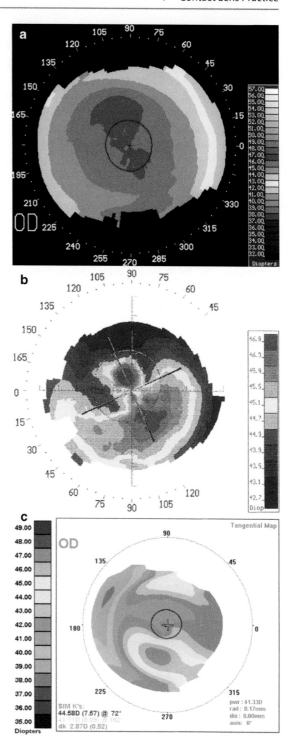

produce an inferior steepening resembling keratoconus. These changes are most easily displayed on a difference map, which subtracts a pre-lens fitting map from the current map (Chap. 5).

After cessation of lens wear, the cornea tends to return to its former shape. The greatest topographic changes occur over the first 1–2 months, but it may take 5 months or more for a normal pattern to return. Some patients appear to stabilise with an abnormal pattern, suggesting that the effect can be irreversible. The topographic changes induced by soft lenses normalise in about 2–5 weeks but can take up to 8 weeks with rigid gas permeable lenses [18, 20].

Some patients with corneal warpage have irregular keratometry mires or a change in their keratometry readings, but for many, the topographic changes can only be detected by computer-assisted videokeratoscopy [21]. This emphasises the importance of obtaining topography prior to refractive surgical procedures in contact lens wearers (Chap. 13). It has been suggested the minimum delay between the removal of contact lenses and the preoperative assessment should be 2 weeks for soft lenses and 4 weeks for hard and RGP lenses [22]. If abnormalities persist after the cessation of lens wear, topography should be repeated at intervals until the corneal shape has normalised or stabilised.

Orthokeratology

Orthokeratology is the practice of fitting progressively flatter tight-fitting rigid contact lenses with the aim of flattening the cornea sufficiently to reduce myopia [23]. Commonly the lenses are worn overnight so the patient can be free of lenses during the day. Although some eyecare practitioners use this technique, it is associated with refractive changes which are small, variable and temporary and may therefore be of only limited clinical value. There is also a relatively high rate of contact lens-related complications, some of which arise from wearing in the closed eye overnight [24–26]. Corneal topography is essential for the evaluation of the safety and efficacy of such procedures, and further studies are awaited.

Preoperative Assessment for Refractive Surgery

Exclusion criteria for refractive surgery include instability of refraction and the presence of underlying corneal pathology (Chap. 13). Both these conditions are more likely in patients wearing contact lenses as they may have lens-induced corneal warpage, or astigmatism which is not adequately corrected by spectacles [21, 27]. The study of optometric records of previous refractions, keratometry or topography is useful in the preoperative assessment, particularly as 50–90% of patients presenting for myopic refractive surgery have worn or tried contact lenses [22, 28].

Patient/Lens Database

Topography systems can be used to store and retrieve patient data and lens information. Some software allows practice management functions to be performed, although they are not designed to replace the patient traditional record card.

A complete contact lens product database is also maintained and regularly updated so that practitioners can find information on any lens without reference to user manuals. However, information designed for the market in one country or continent is not necessarily applicable to others.

Communications software allows topography maps and e-mails to be sent or received worldwide using the Internet. In the future, such link between the practitioner and the production facility may enable customised RGP lenses to be manufactured to a shape determined by the actual corneal topography.

The data collected by the software in topography systems can provide objective feedback to manufacturers and practitioners with the aim of improving lens fitting algorithms and clinical practice.

As corneal topography facilitates the fitting of rigid gas permeable lenses, the current trend of the increasing use of soft lenses due to comfort and convenience might be partially reversed to the advantage of patients' visual performance. If the cost of topography systems can be reduced, their use may become more widespread, and the standard of RGP lens fitting and contact lens practice in general will be enhanced. Topography manufacturers are working towards this by introducing smaller systems with fewer data points, compact equipment with the placido mires and screen integral in one unit, and portable systems (Chap. 3).

References

References Particularly Worth Reading

1. ACLM Industry Statistics – contact lens market. Today; March 28th 1994; 23.
2. Dart JKG. Predisposing factors in microbial keratitis: the significance of contact lens wear. Br J Ophthalmol. 1988;72:926–30.
3. Dart JKG, Stapleton F, Minassian D. Contact lenses and other risk factors in microbial keratitis. Lancet. 1991;338:650–3.
4. Schein OD, Glynn RJ, Poggio EC, Seddon JM, Kenyon KR. The relative risk of ulcerative keratitis among users of daily-wear and extended-wear soft contact lenses: a case-control study. Microbial Keratitis Study Group. N Engl J Med. 1989;321(12):773–8.
5. Poggio EC, Glynn RJ, Schein OD, Seddon JM, Shannon MJ, Scardino VA, Kenyon KR. The incidence of ulcerative keratitis among users of daily-wear and extended-wear soft contact lenses. N Engl J Med. 1989;321:779–83.
6. Stern GA. Contact lens associated bacterial keratitis: past, present, and future. CLAO J. 1998;24(1):52–6.
7. Keay L, Stapleton F, Schein O. Epidemiology of contact lens-related inflammation and microbial keratitis: a 20-year perspective. Eye Contact Lens. 2007;33:346–53.
8. Stone J, Phillips AJ. Contact lenses. London: Butterworths; 1989.
9. Douthwaite WA. Contact lens optics. London: Butterworths; 1987.

10. *Stevenson RWW, Corbett MC, O'Brart DPS, Rosen ES. Corneal topography in contact lens fitting. Eur J Implant Ref Surg. 1995;7(5):305–317.

11. Fredrick S, Wilson G. The relation between eyelid tension, corneal toricity, and age. Invest Ophthalmol Vis Sci. 1983;24:1367–73.

12. Schnider CM, Kennedy L, Mintle L, Carr C, Hnatko T. Comparison of computerised corneal topography device nomogram and topographical fits to trial lens fitting. Invest Ophthalmol Vis Sci. 1995;36(Suppl):1458.

13. Szcotka LB, Capretta DM, Lass JH. Effect of computerised titration on videokeratoscope contact lens fitting. Invest Ophthalmol Vis Sci. 1995;36(Suppl):1458.

14. *Szczota LB, Capretta DM, Lass JH. Clinical evaluation of a computerised topography software method for fitting rigid gas permeable contact lenses. CLAO J. 1995;20:231–235.

15. Szczotka LB. Evaluation of a topographically based contact lens fitting software. Optom Vis Sci. 1997;74:14–9.

16. *Astin CLK, Gartry DS, Steele ADMcG. Contact lens fitting after photorefractive keratectomy. Br J Ophthalmol. 1996;80:597–603.

17. McCarey B, Zurawski C, O'Shea D. Practical aspects of a corneal topography system. CLAO J. 1992;18:248–54.

18. Wang X, McCulley JP, Bowman RW, et al. Time to resolution of contact lens-induced corneal warpage prior to refractive surgery. CLAO J. 2002;28(4):169–71.

19. Ruiz-Montenegro J, Mafra CH, Wilson SE, Jumper JM, Klyce SD, Mendelson EN. Corneal topographic alterations in normal contact lens wearers. Ophthalmology. 1993;100:128–34.

20. *Wilson SE, Lin DTC, Klyce SD, Reidy JJ, Insler MS. Topographic changes in contact lens-induced warpage. Ophthalmology. 1990;97:734–744.

21. *Wilson SE, Klyce SD. Screening for corneal topographic abnormalities before refractive surgery. Ophthalmology. 1994;101:147–152.

22. Corbett MC, O'Brart DPS, Marshall J. Biological and environmental risk factors for regression after photorefractive keratectomy. Ophthalmology. 1996;103:1381–91.

23. Phillips AJ. Orthokeratology – an alternative to excimer laser. J BCLA. 1995;18:65–71.

24. Hsiao CH, Lin HC, Chen YF, Ma DHK, Yeh LK, Tan HY, Huang SCM, Lin KK. Infectious keratitis related to overnight orthokeratology. Cornea. 2005;24:783–8.

25. Tseng CH, Fong CF, Chen WL, Hou YC, Wang IJ, Hu FR. Overnight orthokeratology-associated microbial keratitis. Cornea. 2005;24(7):778–82.

26. Yepes N, Lee SB, Hill V, Ashenhurst M, Saunders PP, Slomovic AR. Infectious keratitis after overnight orthokeratology in Canada. Cornea. 2005;24(7):857–60.

27. Nesburn AB, Bahri S, Salz J, Rabinowitz YS, Maguen E, Hofbauer J, Belin M, Macy JI. Keratoconus detected by videokeratography in candidates for photorefractive keratectomy. J Refract Surg. 1995;11:194–201.

28. Stevenson RWW. Analysis of post-PRK topography maps. Invest Ophthalmol Vis Sci. 1995;36(Suppl):1792.

Corneal Surface Disease

8

Good vision relies upon the cornea being transparent and having a smooth regular surface. Corneal disease often disrupts the normal anatomy and physiology of the cornea, thereby severely reducing the visual performance of the eye. Irregularities of the corneal surface can result from compression by external masses, abnormalities of the epithelium and alterations within the stroma (Table 8.1). With the advent of corneal topography, we can now detect and quantify such changes. These techniques have improved our understanding of the mechanisms by which pathology can produce changes in corneal topography and also offer promise in improving the management of corneal disease.

External Compression

Masses arising around the eye or in the lid can cause pressure on the corneal surface and distort its topography. Such lesions will cause flattening of the globe directly under the area of compression, with steepening of the curvature adjacent to the area of compression (Fig. 8.1).

Central or paracentral compression may be induced by lid lesions such as haemangiomas and large chalazia [1, 2]. In these cases the associated steepening occurs peripherally. More peripheral flattening is induced by masses at or behind the limbus, such as dermoids, or plombs from retinal surgery (Fig. 8.2).

The astigmatic changes produced by these lesions are of particular clinical importance in children. Such unilateral astigmatic changes may result in amblyopia.

© Springer Nature Switzerland AG 2019
M. Corbett et al., *Corneal Topography*,
https://doi.org/10.1007/978-3-030-10696-6_8

Table 8.1 Classification of topographic changes in corneal disease

Site	Examples	Direct effects	Indirect effects
External pressure			
Central/ paracentral	Chalazion	Central flattening	Peripheral steepening
	Lid haemangioma		
Peripheral	Plomb	Peripheral flattening	Central steepening
	Dermoid		
Tear film			
Deficiency	Keratoconjunctivitis sicca	Focal flattening	–
		Widespread irregularity	
Poor quality	Blepharitis	Artefacts	–
Epithelium			
General irregularity	Corneal oedema	Irregularity	–
	Band keratopathy	Artefacts	
Local depressions	Ulcers	Focal flattening	–
	Dellen	Irregularity	
Local elevations	Pterygium	Focal steepening	–
	Salzmann's nodules	Irregularity	
	Nebulae		
	Thygeson's keratitis		
Stroma			
Local swelling	Herpetic keratitis	Focal steepening	–
Central/ paracentral thinning	Deep corneal ulcers	Focal flattening	Adjacent steepening
Peripheral thinning	Terrien's degeneration	<u>Mild/moderate</u>	Steepening perpendicularly
	Mooren's ulcer	Flattening in affected meridian	
	Peripheral gutters in systemic disease	Severe	Complex
	Pellucid degeneration	Ectasia and steepening	
Ectasia	Keratoconus	Central steepening	–
	Keratoglobus		
	Pellucid degeneration		

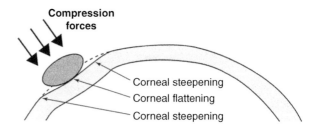

Fig. 8.1 External compression. Masses around the eye cause flattening directly under the area of compression, with steepening in adjacent areas

Compression forces

Corneal steepening
Corneal flattening
Corneal steepening

Fig. 8.2 Radial plomb.
After retinal detachment
surgery, a radial plomb
sutured 4 mm posterior to
the limbus in the 75°
meridian caused flattening
of the sclera beneath the
plomb and steepening of
the adjacent cornea

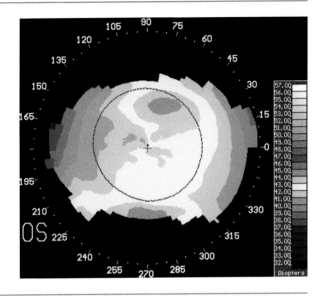

Tear Film Disturbances

Corneal topography devices, whether utilising reflection or projection, image the
air-tear fluid interface. Therefore, corneal topography is influenced by abnormalities in either the quantity or the quality of tears or their distribution across the corneal surface [3–6].

Primary anomalies of the tear film may be the result of a wide variety of systemic and local disorders. Tear fluid deficiency in conditions such as keratoconjunctivitis sicca leads to focal patches of drying which appear as localised areas
of flattening (Fig. 6.5). An altered tear fluid composition can also interfere with
the analysis of the captured image. For example, excessive oil in the tear fluid
can appear as dark swirls on a videokeratograph and prevent detection of the
position of the mires (Fig. 6.6). In both these situations, the patient should be
asked to blink immediately before capture of the image. Tear film abnormalities
can also exacerbate surface irregularity by causing epithelial cell degradation
and death [7].

Epithelial Disease

An intact, healthy corneal epithelial surface with a normal, smooth tear film is
essential for the regular refraction of light by the eye and the formation of a clear
retinal image. Any disturbances in this surface will result in a degradation of the
corneal topography and seriously impair visual performance [8, 9]. Such anomalies
may be localised or may diffusely involve the entire corneal surface. Their effect on
vision is dependent primarily upon their location rather than the total area affected.

Surface irregularities over the visual axis, however small, will profoundly disturb visual function. In contrast, larger abnormalities towards the periphery will have less effect.

By quantifying the irregularity of the corneal surface (Chap. 5), topography can help determine the proportion of the visual loss which is attributable to irregular astigmatism as opposed to loss of corneal transparency. If visual disturbance is principally due to disruption of surface topography, then rigid contact lenses may improve the visual acuity to acceptable levels. If loss of corneal transparency is primarily responsible for visual loss, then keratoplasty is usually necessary for visual rehabilitation.

Corneal topography can sometimes detect subtle epithelial abnormalities which are not necessarily revealed by biomicroscopic slit lamp examination. Visual disturbance in patients with minor central epithelial irregularity is usually due to changes in surface topography. For example, patients with recurrent epithelial erosion syndrome may complain of significant visual symptoms, despite an entirely normal appearance on slit lamp examination. However, videokeratoscopy can detect the subtle abnormalities in the surface topography which reveal the underlying epithelial abnormality (Fig. 8.3).

In patients with a poor tear film or marked surface irregularity, topography is most accurately measured by devices utilising projection methods rather than reflection (Chap. 3). In these situations, techniques such as keratometry and videokeratoscopy have three major limitations [10, 11]. Firstly, they require an intact tear film to provide a reflective surface on which the image of the mires is generated. Secondly, if irregularities have a small periodicity, the individual rings of the mires cannot be identified. Thirdly, if irregularities have a slightly larger periodicity, the rings can be identified, but the algorithms are inadequate to accurately reconstruct the details of the surface. In the latter situation, local radius of curvature is more accurate than global radius of curvature (Chap. 1).

Aetiology

There are numerous disorders affecting the corneal epithelium that can cause topographical irregularities. These can result from a multitude of inflammatory or noninflammatory processes which may be a consequence of both localised ocular pathology and more widespread systemic disease. Such processes may be confined to the epithelium itself or involve the tear fluid, underlying corneal stroma [12], or adjacent ocular structures.

Mechanisms

Whatever the aetiology of the corneal disease, the epithelium responds in a limited number of ways: loss, thinning, hyperplasia, metaplasia, oedema, basement membrane changes and accumulation of excessive or abnormal material. These processes may be generalised or localised.

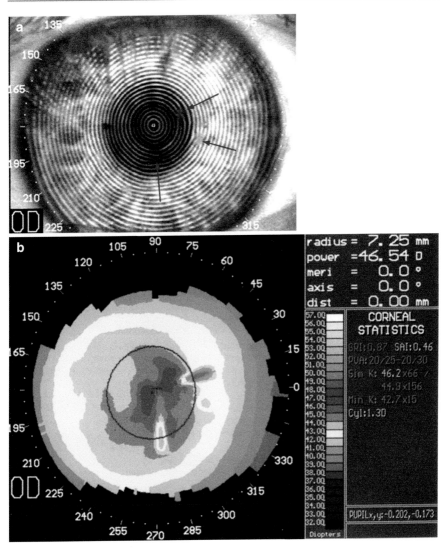

Fig. 8.3 Recurrent erosion. In this patient with recurrent corneal erosion syndrome, no epithelial abnormality could be detected on biomicroscopic examination between attacks. (**a**) The videokeratograph showed irregularity of the mires (arrows) in the 10°, 270° and 350° semimeridians, about 1–2 mm from the corneal centre. (**b**) These correspond to areas of focal flattening on the topography

Epithelial abnormalities not only have a direct effect on the shape of the corneal surface, but they also influence the distribution of the overlying tear fluid. Localised drying can occur in areas where the epithelial cells are sick or damaged, leading to greater disruption of the surface topography [13] (Fig. 8.4). In contrast, the tear fluid can sometimes help to smooth the topography over epithelial irregularities. It tends to pool in surface depressions and become thinner over protuberances. This explains

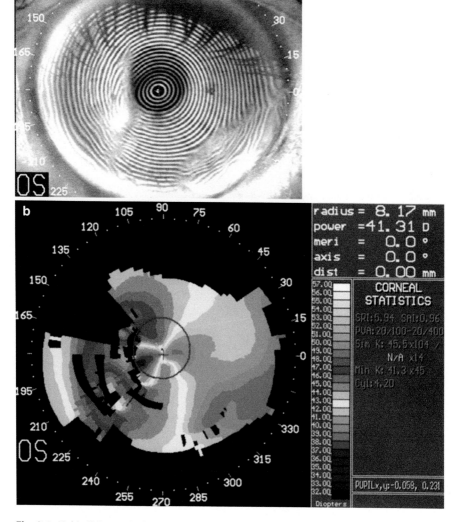

Fig. 8.4 Epithelial metaplasia. The epithelial irregularity and associated tear film disturbance is most marked nasally. In this area the videokeratoscopy rings (**a**) merge into one another. They cannot be distinguished well enough for the topography (**b**) to be reconstructed accurately, and many data points are missing (the black areas)

why some patients with surface irregularity report improved vision after blinking, when the cornea is resurfaced by tear fluid. Similarly, the application of a hard contact lens can improve visual acuity by providing a smooth anterior refracting surface.

The corneal epithelium is also influenced by the underlying superficial corneal stroma [12]. Like the tear film, it tends to be thicker over local depressions and thinner over protuberances. Therefore, in the same way, the epithelium can help to smooth the surface over localised stromal irregularities. In contrast, there are also situations in which the epithelium is unhealthy over a stromal defect, such as a neurotrophic ulcer. In this case the epithelium contributes to the irregularity of the topography.

It can therefore be seen that the shape of the corneal surface is determined by a complex interaction between the tear fluid, epithelium and superficial stroma. The resultant topographical patterns can be extremely irregular, non-specific and difficult to evaluate.

Generalised Irregularity

Generalised epithelial irregularity, whether due to oedema, metaplasia, deposition or other pathologies, usually causes a non-specific disruption of the surface topography (Fig. 8.4).

Local Depressions

Local depressions in the corneal surface, for example, as a result of a small corneal ulcer (Figs. 2.6 and 8.5) or dellen, cause a localised area of corneal flattening.

Local Elevations

Local elevations of the corneal surface include Salzmann's nodules, proud nebulae (Figs. 4.2 and 4.5) and Thygeson's superficial punctate keratitis. These cause focal steepening [14].

Pterygia

Pterygia are an excellent example of a structural abnormality occurring at the level of the epithelium, which also influences the overlying tear film and the underlying stroma.

It has long been accepted that pterygia tend to produce corneal astigmatism. However, the nature and extent of astigmatism that may be induced are the subject of some debate. Early work using keratometry to study the effect of small pterygia found a predominance of horizontal steepening [15]. Others found horizontal flattening to be more frequent, although the incidence was not significantly different from age-matched controls [16].

It has since been confirmed using corneal topography that eyes with pterygia often have irregular astigmatism, with the flattest axis within 20° of the horizontal [17–19] (Fig. 8.6). The average induced topographic astigmatism is about 4D and can be as high as 10D. However, the refractive astigmatism is usually less marked, and the vision often remains good until the pterygium encroaches on the pupillary zone [20] (Fig. 8.7).

Pterygia can potentially induce horizontal flattening by two mechanisms (Fig. 8.8). Firstly, the tear meniscus in front of the head of the pterygium fills in the angle between the pterygium and the paracentral cornea. Secondly, the pterygium may be having a direct effect on the underlying stroma. It is unlikely that forces applied by fibrovascular contractile elements within the pterygium have a major effect, as they

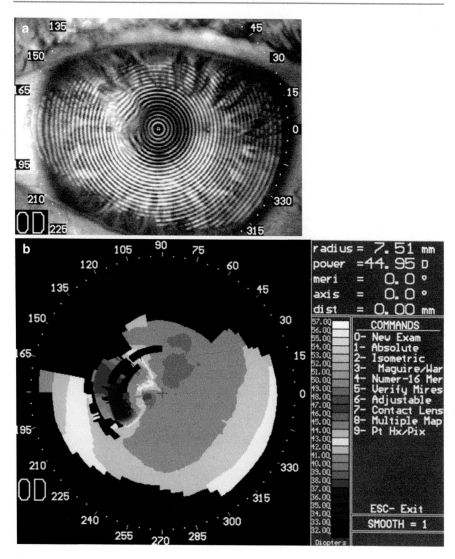

Fig. 8.5 Infectious keratitis. A localised depression of the superotemporal paracentral cornea (**a**) caused focal flattening and irregularity (**b**)

would be expected to steepen the cornea (in a similar manner to a tight suture). Possibly changes in the anterior stroma beneath the pterygium have a role. Other perilimbal lesions such as dermoids can produce similar topographical effects.

Management

The development of clinical excimer lasers in the mid-1980s has offered a new approach to the treatment of superficial corneal pathologies [21]. The

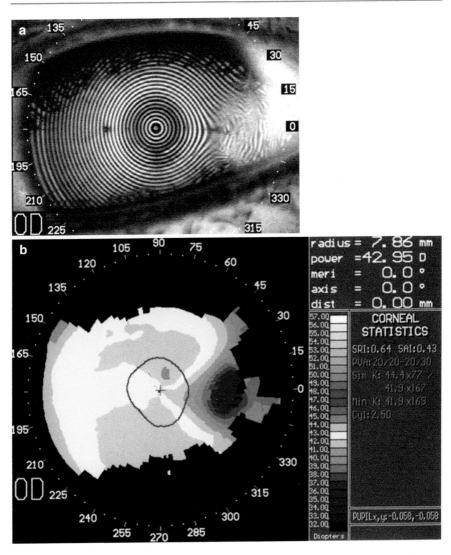

Fig. 8.6 Moderate pterygium. The pterygium has encroached about 2.5 mm onto the nasal cornea (**a**), but the predicted visual acuity remains good because the associated flattening is restricted to the peripheral and paracentral cornea, leaving only mild regular astigmatism within the pupillary aperture (**b**)

advantages of such lasers are derived from two unique characteristics. The first is their ability to remove corneal tissue with extreme precision and minimal collateral damage (Chap. 13). The second is the large diameter of their beams, typically several millimetres in diameter, allowing the simultaneous treatment of wide areas. With excimer laser technology, it is now possible to remove unwanted tissue and precisely resculpture the anterior cornea to create a new optical surface.

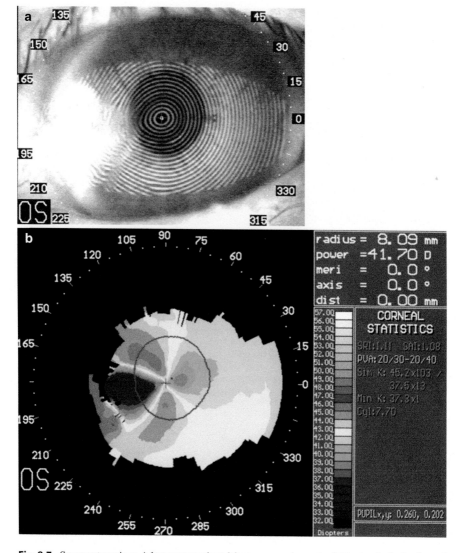

Fig. 8.7 Severe pterygium. A larger pterygium (**a**) causes much greater flattening in the horizontal nasal semimeridian (**b**) and induces a greater degree of with-the-rule astigmatism (>6DC). There is associated steepening in the adjacent meridian

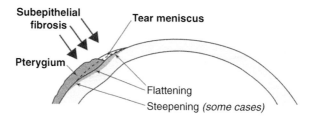

Fig. 8.8 Pterygium mechanisms. Pterygia can induce horizontal flattening by two mechanisms. First, the tear meniscus fills in the angle at the head of the pterygium. Second, subepithelial fibrosis beneath the head of the pterygium can cause localised flattening, with steepening of the adjacent cornea

Topography maps have been used to plan excimer laser photoablative treatments to correct irregular astigmatism [22]. Steep areas on the corneal maps were identified and then "flattened" using small diameter excimer laser ablations. This selective flattening was aimed at minimising the differences between steeper and flatter geographical areas within the optical zone of the cornea, to improve the refractive performance of the eye. However, to flatten a steep slope, tissue must be removed from the top of the slope, but not the bottom. It is therefore more appropriate to use elevation maps for this purpose, so that tissue can be removed from the highest areas, rather than the steepest areas.

These techniques will hopefully improve the visual rehabilitation of patients with extensive corneal pathology by reducing their dependence upon rigid contact lenses and avoiding ocular surgery.

References

*References Particularly Worth Reading

1. Plager DA, Snyder SK. Resolution of astigmatism after surgical resection of capillary hemangiomas in infants. Ophthalmology. 1997;104:1102–6.
2. Park YM, Lee JS. The effects of chalazion excision on corneal surface aberrations. Cont Lens Anterior Eye. 2014;37(5):342–5.
3. Mishima S. Some physiological aspects of the precorneal tearfilm. Arch Ophthalmol. 1965;73:233.
4. Pavlopoulos GP, Horn J, Feldman ST. The effect of artificial tears on computer-assisted corneal topography in normal eyes and after penetrating keratoplasty. Am J Ophthalmol. 1995;119:712–22.
5. *Novak KD, Kohnen T, Chang-Godinich A, Soper BA, Kennedy P, Wang Q, Padrick T, Koch DD. Changes in computerised videokeratography induced by artificial tears. J Cat Refract Surg. 1997;23:1023–1028.
6. Szczotka-Flynn L. Ocular surface influences on corneal topography. Ocul Surf. 2004;2(3):188–200.
7. Bron AJ, Mengher LS. The ocular surface in keratoconjunctivitis sicca. Eye. 1989;3:428–37.
8. Dierick HG, Missotten L. Is the corneal contour influenced by a tension in the superficial epithelial cells? A new hypothesis. Refract Corneal Surg. 1992;8:54–9.
9. Montés-Micó R, Cervino A, Ferrer-Blasco T. The tear film and the optical quality of the eye. Ocul Surf. 2010;8(4):185–92.
10. Sanders RD, Gills JP, Martin RG. When keratometric measurements do not accurately reflect corneal topography. J Cat Refract Surg. 1993;19(Suppl):131–5.
11. Varssano D, Rapuano CJ, Luchs JI. Comparison of keratometric values of healthy and diseased eyes measured by Javal keratometer, EyeSys and PAR. J Cat Refract Surg. 1997;23:419–22.
12. Geggel HS. Effect of peripheral subepithelial fibrosis on corneal transplant topography. J Cat Refract Surg. 1996;22:135–8.
13. Cui X, Hong J, Wang F, et al. Assessment of corneal epithelial thickness in dry eye patients. Optom Vis Sci. 2014;91(12):1446–54.
14. Maharana PK, Sharma N, Das S, et al. Salzmann's nodular degeneration. Ocul Surf. 2016;14(1):20–30.
15. Forsius H, Eriksson A. Pterygium and its relation to arcus senelis, pinguecula and other similar conditions. Acta Ophthalmol. 1962;40:402–10.
16. Hansen A, Norn M. Astigmatism and surface phenomenon in pterygium. Acta Ophthalmol. 1980;58:174–81.
17. *Pavilack MA, Halpern BL. Corneal topographic changes induced by pterygia. J Refract Surg. 1995;11:92–95.

18. Oldenberg JB, Garbus J, McDonnell JM, McDonnell PJ. Conjunctival pterygia. Mechanism of topographic changes. Cornea. 1990;9:200–4.
19. *O'Brart DPS, Corbett MC, Rosen ES. The topography of corneal disease. Eur J Implant Ref Surg. 1995;7 (3): 173–183.
20. Bedrossian RH. The effect of pterygium surgery on refraction and curvature. Arch Ophthalmol. 1960;64:105–9.
21. O'Brart DPS, Gartry DS, Lohmann C, Patmore A, Kerr Muir MG, Marshall J. Treatment of band keratopathy by excimer laser phototherapeutic keratectomy (PTK): surgical techniques and long-term follow-up. Br J Ophthalmol. 1993;77:702–8.
22. Gibralter R, Trokel SL. Correction of irregular astigmatism with the excimer laser. Ophthalmology. 1994;101:1310–5.

Stromal Disease

9

As with the superficial cornea, stromal disease may be the result of a wide variety of inflammatory and noninflammatory disorders, with either local or systemic origins. Disease of the corneal stroma induces topographic changes as a result of swelling, thinning or stretching (ectasia) (Table 8.1). The resulting patterns are more specific than those resulting from superficial corneal disease (Table 9.1). They are determined by the site, size and depth of the area involved.

Mechanisms

Direct Effects

Stromal disease has a direct effect on corneal topography at the site of the pathology, in the same manner as superficial corneal disease. This may cause either local steepening or local flattening.

Adjacent Effects

Irregularities of the stroma may be larger than those affecting the surface, and therefore they can influence the topography of the adjacent area. For example, there may be local steepening at the edge of an area of thinning or local flattening surrounding an elevation.

Table 9.1 Features of the topographic changes in superficial corneal and stromal disease.

Superficial corneal disease	Stromal disease
Non-specific topographic changes	More specific topographic patterns
Direct effect on topography	Widespread and distant effects
May be self-limiting	More likely to be prolonged or permanent
Good visual improvements with hard contact lenses	Less easily corrected by hard contact lenses

© Springer Nature Switzerland AG 2019
M. Corbett et al., *Corneal Topography*,
https://doi.org/10.1007/978-3-030-10696-6_9

Distant Effects

Stromal lesions, especially thinning, can also affect the topography of areas of "normal" cornea, distant from the site of pathology. When this phenomenon occurs as a result of incisional refractive surgery, it is termed "coupling". The mechanisms involved are best explained by first considering the structure [1] and biomechanics [2–5] of the normal cornea.

The cornea forms part of the tough outer coat of the eye and therefore has a role in maintaining the intraocular pressure, supporting the intraocular structures and resisting trauma and infection. The stroma is the layer which provides the necessary mechanical strength. It contains densely packed collagen lamellae which arch from limbus to limbus in layers parallel to the corneal surface. X-ray diffraction studies by Meek et al. have shown the anterior lamellae are highly interwoven and randomly directed when observed en face [6], whereas the posterior lamellae appear to have preferred inferior-superior or nasal-temporal orientation [7]. The exception to this is deep in the corneal periphery where a ring of fibres runs circumferentially. Studies also suggest the presence of a network of collagen lamellae that originate in the adjacent sclera and enter the cornea close to the inferior, superior, nasal and temporal positions [8]. There is mirror symmetry between both eyes, and these peripheral collagen fibrils appear to have a larger diameter to those in the central cornea [9].

Between the collagen fibres, the extracellular matrix is rich in glycosaminoglycans, which are large molecules with a high viscosity and elasticity. The compact, regular structure of the stroma is fundamental to the maintenance of a normal corneal shape. It is thought this is maintained by a balance between the expansive force of osmotic pressure and the attractive force between glycosaminoglycans and the collagen fibrils [10].

Bowman's layer is the relatively acellular anterior 8–14 μm of the superficial corneal stroma [1]. Its mechanical properties do not differ from those of the remaining stroma [4].

When damage to the stroma occurs, the stability of the corneal shape is compromised. Defects in stromal collagen lamellae, whether caused by surgical incisions, loss of tissue or thinning, cause new stress equilibria to be set up in the cornea [3]. Meek et al. have shown inter- and intra-collagen lamellar displacement and slippage leading to thinning and associated change in corneal curvature in patients with keratoconus [11]. The region of greatest thinning was elongated vertically and contained the least aligned collagen.

The induced changes in corneal shape are most easily seen when there are single, deep focal areas of thinning. In general, this causes flattening of the corneal curvature along the meridian perpendicular to the tangent of the stromalthinning.

The mechanisms by which loss of peripheral stromal tissue can cause central corneal flattening are not fully understood. The destruction of lamellae running across the cornea from limbus to limbus may allow stretching and relaxation of the peripheral corneal tissues. Such structural changes may cause the peripheral cornea to "bow" outwards, resulting in flattening of the central cornea [5].

Coupling effects produce steepening in the meridian perpendicular to the flattening. These are likely to result from the presence of intact rings of lamellae running

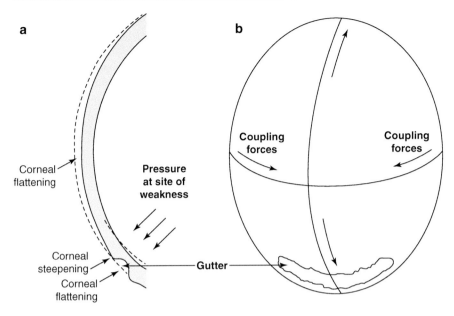

Fig. 9.1 Peripheral gutter mechanism. Destruction of collagen lamellae by a peripheral gutter can cause outward bowing of the weakened area due to the force of the intraocular pressure (**a**). This causes flattening of the central cornea. The intact circumferential lamellae around the base of the cornea are stretched and become oval. These forces are transmitted to the perpendicular meridian where they cause compression forces and steepening as a result of coupling (**b**). In addition, there may be local steepening and flattening over the edges and base of the gutter (**a**)

circumferentially around the base of the cornea. Presumably the flattening in the pathological axis stretches the rings until they become oval. The resultant compressive forces would then be transmitted to the radial fibres in the perpendicular axis, which would therefore steepen (Fig. 9.1).

Topographic Patterns

The exact topographic pattern induced will depend on the site, size and depth of the stromal loss or swelling and in particular whether the pathology is located centrally or in the corneal periphery. Other factors which influence the topographic changes are pressure from the upper lid and the presence or absence of secondary epithelial and tear film disturbances.

Stromal Swelling

Stromal swelling is often the result of oedema, which is a non-specific response to injury. In the presence of intact collagen lamellae anteriorly, diffuse oedema (e.g.

following endothelial damage) induces very little change in the overall shape of the anterior corneal surface. In this situation, the stromal swelling is directed posteriorly, resulting in folds in Descemet's membrane [12].

Stromal swelling may project anteriorly if it is associated with damage to the superficial collagen lamellae or the generation of new wound healing material (e.g. herpes simplex disciform keratitis). In this situation the affected area is steepened and may demonstrate irregularities (Fig. 9.2).

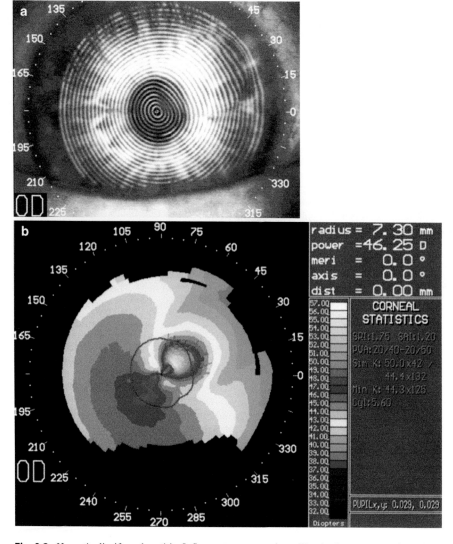

Fig. 9.2 Herpetic disciform keratitis. Inflammatory stromal swelling in the superonasal quadrant (**a**) has caused focal corneal steepening with more peripheral flattening (**b**)

Central and Paracentral Thinning

Small degrees of central or paracentral thinning produce a localised area of corneal flattening or irregularity in a similar manner to that described for corneal surface disease (Chap. 8). When the thinning is of moderate depth, the flattened area may be surrounded by area of steepening relating to the edge of the lesion (e.g. ulcerative keratitis).

Deeper defects can compromise the stability of the cornea and result in steepening at distant sites (Fig. 9.3). In cases of very advanced tissue loss, there may be anterior protrusion at the site of the lesion, with the formation of a descemetocele. As this extreme thinning occurs, the topography reverses, and the affected area becomes steeper than the surrounding area.

Thinning of the central cornea, particularly if associated with irregularity, can significantly reduce visual function. Most cases are not correctable by spectacles but require rigid contact lenses. In those with marked irregularity or corneal opacification, keratoplasty may be required.

Peripheral Thinning

Loss of peripheral corneal stroma usually results in flattening of the central cornea in the same meridian [13–15]. This is commonly associated with steepening of the perpendicular meridian as a result of coupling (Fig. 9.4).

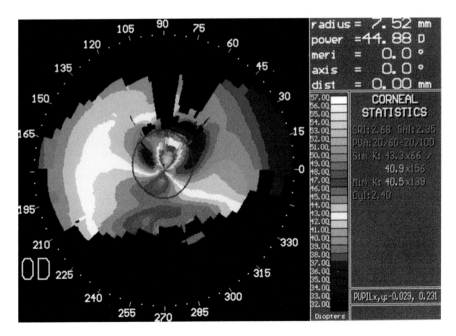

Fig. 9.3 Corneal ulcer. Healed infectious keratitis causing a localised depression in the superior paracentral cornea. In this area the videokeratoscopy rings are more widely spaced (Fig. 2.6), and the colour shows focal flattening. The ulcer was deep enough to erode superficial collagen lamellae, and this lead to steepening of the opposite semimeridian

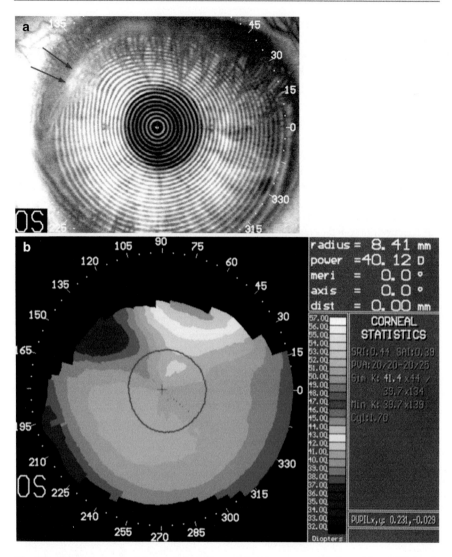

Fig. 9.4 Terrien's marginal degeneration. The peripheral gutter extends from 90 to 170° (partly obscured by the upper lid). (**a**) The videokeratoscopy mires are blurred over the gutter itself (arrows), preventing reconstruction of its topography by this technique. This can be overcome by using techniques that utilise the Scheimpflug principle (see Chap. 4). (**b**) However, the colour-coded map shows that the gutter has produced local flattening superonasally where it is deepest and steeping in the orthogonal meridian. The central cornea within the pupillary aperture is relatively unaffected and therefore the predicted visual acuity remains good

If thinning progresses, peripheral gutters can extend circumferentially or even centrally. As a greater circumference is flattened, the steep meridian becomes closer together producing an "arching bow tie" pattern (Fig. 9.5). If ectasia develops there may be a more generalised steepening of the central cornea (Fig. 9.6). With more extensive stromal tissue destruction, the vector forces become increasingly complicated, and the topographic changes are more difficult to predict.

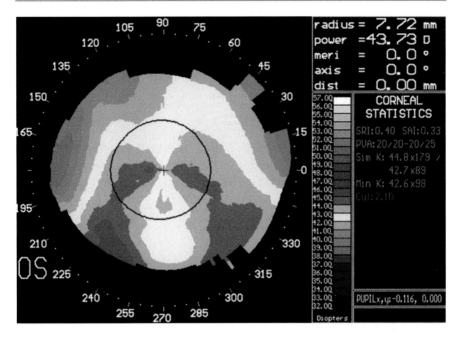

Fig. 9.5 Pellucid marginal degeneration. More extensive peripheral guttering leads to irregular astigmatism, such as this arching bow tie pattern. The less severely affected right eye is shown in Fig. 5.11c

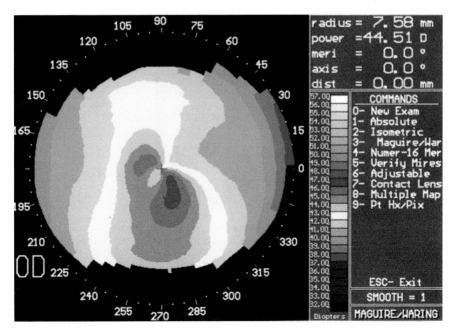

Fig. 9.6 Pellucid marginal degeneration with ectasia. If guttering becomes more severe, ectasia may occur, leading to generalised steepening of the central or inferior cornea

In peripheral stromal thinning, corneal topography is often spherocylindrical and can be corrected by spectacle lenses until the later stages. When extensive thinning and ectasia occur, scleral lenses may be required. Keratoplasty is often difficult due to the involvement of the peripheral cornea.

Ectasia

Thinning and stretching of the corneal stroma can result in it protruding forward. This may occur secondary to the processes described above or as a primary event in keratoconus, keratoglobus and possibly pellucid marginal degeneration [16]. The topography of these conditions has been studied in depth, and is described in Chap. 11.

Trauma

Partial- or full-thickness penetration of the corneal stroma can result in a variety of topographic appearances depending upon not only the site and size of the lesion but also its age and treatment. Stromal oedema can cause localised steepening (Fig. 9.7), whereas overtightening of sutures may cause focal flattening with adjacent steepening.

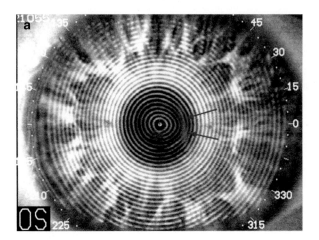

Fig. 9.7 Penetrating corneal injury. A 1.5 mm full-thickness linear perforation (arrows) 1 mm temporal to the visual axis (**a**) causing localised corneal steepening and irregularity (**b**)

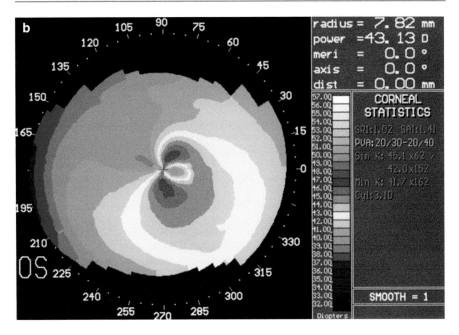

Fig. 9.7 (continued)

References

*References Particularly Worth Reading

1. Hogan MJ, Alvorado JA, Weddell JE. The cornea. In: Histology of the human eye: an atlas and textbook. Philadelphia: Saunders; 1971.
2. Buzard KA. Biomechanics of the cornea – who needs it? [editorial]. Refract Corneal Surg. 1992;8:125–6.
3. *Buzard KA. Introduction to biomechanics of the cornea [review]. Refract Corneal Surg. 1992;8:126–138.
4. Seiler T, Matallana M, Sendler S, Bende T. Does Bowman's layer determine the biomechanical properties of the cornea? Refract Corneal Surg. 1992;8:139–42.
5. Buzard KA, Ronk JF, Friedlander MH, Tepper DJ, Hoeltzel DA, Choe K-I. Quantitative measurement of wound spreading in radial keratotomy. Refract Corneal Surg. 1992;8:217–23.
6. Abahussin M, Hayes S, Knox Cartwright NE, et al. 3D collagen orientation study in human cornea using X-ray diffraction and femtosecond laser technology. Invest Ophthalmol Vis Sci. 2009;50:5159–64.

7. Kamma-Lorger CS, Boote C, Hayes S, et al. Collagen and mature elastic fibre organisation as a function of depth in the human cornea and limbus. J Struct Biol. 2010;169:424–30.
8. *Meek KM, Knupp C. Corneal structure and transparency. Prog Retin Eye Res. 2015;49:1–16.
9. Boote C, Kamma-Lorger CS, Hayes S, et al. Quantification of collagen organisation in the peripheral human cornea at micron-scale resolution. Biophys J. 2011;101:33–42.
10. *Lewis PN, Pinali C, Young RD, et al. Structural interactions between collagen and proteoglycans are elucidated by three-dimensional electron tomography of bovine cornea. Structure. 2010;18:23–245.
11. *Meek KM, Tuft SJ, Huang Y, et al. Changes in collagen orientation and distribution in keratoconus corneas. Invest Ophthalmol Vis Sci. 2005;46(6):1948–56.
12. Ousley PJ, Terry MA. Hydration effects on corneal topography. Arch Ophthalmol. 1996;114:181–5.
13. *Wilson SE, Lin DTC, Klyce SD, Insler MS. Terrien's marginal degeneration: corneal topography. Refract Corneal Surg. 1990;6:15–20.
14. *Rumelt S, Rehany U. Computerized corneal topography of furrow corneal degeneration. J Cat Refract Surg. 1997;23:856–859.
15. *Corbett MC, O'Brart DPS, Stultiens BATh, Jongsma FHM, Marshall J. Corneal topography using a new moiré image-based system. Eur J Implant Ref Surg. 1995;7:353–370.
16. *Karabatsas CH, Cook SD. Topographic analysis in pellucid marginal degeneration and keratoglobus. Eye. 1996;10:451–455.

Corneal Ectasia

10

The primary corneal ectasias are a group of noninflammatory diseases in which the cornea protrudes forwards as a result of stromal thinning. The three conditions in this group are keratoconus, keratoglobus and pellucid marginal degeneration. There is considerable overlap between their clinical features, and they may even co-exist in an individual or in the same family. Differentiation may be made between them on the basis of the site of the stromal thinning. In keratoconus the thinning is paracentral and occurs most commonly below the horizontal. The thinning is in the inferior periphery in pellucid marginal degeneration (Fig. 9.6) and is generalised in keratoglobus.

By far the most common of these conditions is keratoconus. Its topography has been studied extensively, and therefore it will be used as the main example in this chapter. Corneal topography has roles in both the diagnosis and management of keratoconus and its related conditions (Table 10.1).

Clinical Features of Keratoconus

Keratoconus typically presents in adolescence and progresses until the third or fourth decade. It is a bilateral, asymmetrical condition that is usually sporadic, but 8–10% of cases have a hereditary component and family history, often with an autosomal dominant mode of inheritance with variable expressivity [1–9].

Aetiology

The precise aetiology of keratoconus is not fully understood with several different biochemical, physical and genetic pathways implicated. It can occur as an isolated condition or in association with ocular and systemic disorders such as atopy, vernal disease, Down's syndrome and connective tissue disorders such as Marfan's

© Springer Nature Switzerland AG 2019   147
M. Corbett et al., *Corneal Topography*,
https://doi.org/10.1007/978-3-030-10696-6_10

Table 10.1 Role of corneal topography in the diagnosis and management of keratoconus

Role of topography in keratoconus	
Diagnosis	Detection of subclinical disease
	Screening before refractive surgery
	Genetic studies
	Differential diagnosis
	Keratoglobus
	Pellucid marginal degeneration
	Contact lens-induced corneal warpage
	Decentration of refractive procedures
	Classification
	Severity
	Location
	Shape
Management	Monitor disease progression
	Contact lens fitting
	Penetrating keratoplasty
	Preoperative assessment
	Postoperative management

syndrome [10]. It can be associated with eye rubbing and allergic eye disease, but the evidence does not show whether this is causative or a confounding factor [11–13]. There is also an association with apical touch of rigid gas permeable contact lenses, but no evidence of which is cause or effect [ref].

Epidemiology
Recent evidence suggests the annual incidence and prevalence may be much higher than previously thought: Godefrooij et al. conducted an epidemiological study looking at 4.4 million patients in the Netherlands and found the annual incidence was 1:7500 (13.3 cases per 100,000) and the estimated prevalence was 1:375 (265 cases per 100,000) [14]. These figures are five- to tenfold higher than previously reported in population studies. This is thought to be due to a combination of earlier detection by using more sensitive topographic measurements and more comprehensive data collection.

Clinical Signs
In the past the diagnosis of keratoconus has relied upon the history and the subjective assessment of clinical signs. Patients often present with a history of progressive myopia, oblique astigmatism and a reduction of spectacle-corrected visual acuity. In some, optometrists noticed an "oil droplet" reflex on direct ophthalmoscopy or "scissoring" of the retinoscopy reflex. The detection of keratoconus was one of the most frequent indications for using a handheld Placido disc. In advanced disease the clinical features are usually obvious and include thinning and scarring

of the central and inferior cornea, Vogt's striae (vertical stress lines visible in the deep stroma) and Fleischer's ring (epithelial iron deposition line) around the base of the cone.

Subclinical Keratoconus

In early disease these features may not be obvious. The detection of ectasia has been greatly improved with the advent of corneal topography and particularly digital analysis such as the superior/inferior ratio (S:I), keratoconus prediction index (KPI) and screening programmes such as the Belin-Ambrosio Enhanced Ectasia Display (BAD).

As the border between normality and keratoconus has become blurred, it has now appeared that the condition is more common than previously thought and has a wider spectrum. Family members of patients with keratoconus may have subclinical disease or other forms of ectasia (keratoglobus or pellucid marginal degeneration) [3]. However, prospective analysis and documentation of more cases are required to determine the clinical significance of these early cones.

The detection of subclinical keratoconus has assumed greater significance with the development and expansion of refractive surgery over recent years [4–6, 44, 45]. There have been three main concerns regarding the treatment of eyes with subclinical disease. Firstly, instability of the preoperative refraction and postoperative progression of the disease can reduce the long-term accuracy of refractive procedures. Secondly, it has been postulated that a degree of tectonic weakening of the cornea induced by radial keratotomy and other incisional procedures may accelerate the development and progression of clinically significant disease. Thirdly, eyes with keratoconus may have an abnormal wound healing response which could result in excessive regression, irregular astigmatism or haze. Whilst there is evidence eyes with subclinical (or Forme Fruste) keratoconus may not be associated with these problems [46–48], it is widely accepted that laser refractive surgery in such cases may be contraindicated.

Up to 8% of myopes presenting for refractive surgery have features suspicious of keratoconus on topographic analysis [44]. However, by excluding those with instability of refraction, reduced spectacle-corrected visual acuity, myopia >10.00D and astigmatism >2.00D, this can be reduced to 1–2% [49]. In patients with high astigmatism, especially if oblique, the number of cases with subclinical keratoconus increases to 10–20%.

Topographic Features

In keratoconus, the thinning most commonly occurs just inferior to the corneal centre. Protrusion in this region gives the corneal surface an exaggerated prolate shape. The point of maximum protrusion is termed the apex of the cone. It is the highest point of the cornea and therefore has a slope of zero (in the same way as the very top

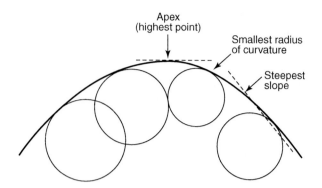

Fig. 10.1 Structure of a cone. The apex of the cone in keratoconus is at the highest point of the cornea and can therefore only be located from height or slope maps. The circles represent the relative radius of curvature of different parts of the cornea. For eccentric cones, the smallest radius of curvature (greatest power) is peripheral to the apex. The region of steepest slope may be even more peripheral. Therefore it is important to appreciate which scale is used in any map studied

of a hill is horizontal). The points of maximum steepness and greatest power (or smallest radius of curvature) are usually both inferior to the apex (Fig. 10.1). This results in astigmatism, which is asymmetric between the upper and lower hemispheres of the cornea.

Keratoscopy

In keratoconus, the videokeratoscopy mires are distorted and tend to be oval. For an inferior cone, they lie closest together in the inferocentral region, where the cornea is steepest, and furthest apart superiorly, where the cornea is flattest [15, 16] (Figs. 5.2a, 10.2a and 10.3a). Such Placido disc images are useful in the detection of moderate or severe keratoconus, but when viewed alone, they provide no quantitative information, so very mild cases could be missed.

In cases of severe keratoconus, particularly those with surface irregularities such as proud nebulae, the keratoscopy mires are distorted and can merge into one another (Figs. 5.2a and 10.3a). However, this qualitative information can be useful in understanding the patient's symptoms. Videokeratoscopes require a smooth intact tear film to produce a clear reflected image of the mires, which can be detected and analysed. Any disturbance in the air-tear-epithelial interface will cause degradation of the mire pattern resulting in a reduction in the quality and quantity of topographic information that can be obtained from it. More useful information can be obtained from irregular or non-reflective corneas by systems utilising the principle of projection, rather than those dependent upon reflection [17, 18] (Chap. 5).

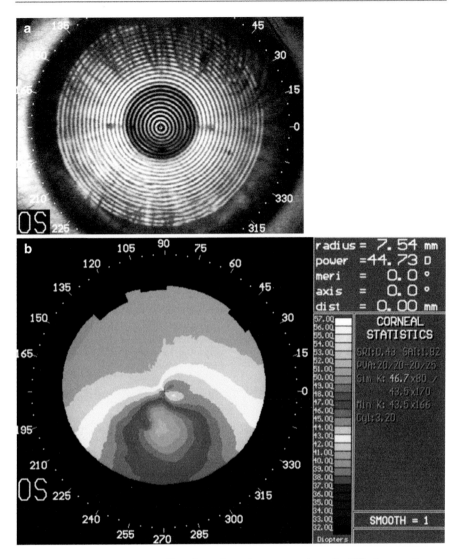

Fig. 10.2 Moderate keratoconus. Even in moderate keratoconus, it can be difficult to see the narrowing between the rings inferiorly on the videokeratograph (**a**). However, it is obvious form the colour-coded map (**b**) that there is corneal steepening in this region

Topographic Maps

In established keratoconus, the topography map shows localised steepening associated with the area of the cone, with corresponding flattening in the opposite hemisphere [23, 24]. There is usually displacement of the corneal apex towards the direction of the cone, which is where the cornea is thinnest (Fig. 10.4).

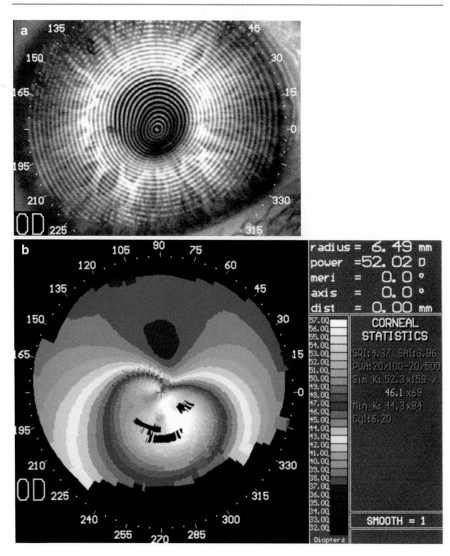

Fig. 10.3 Severe keratoconus. In more severe cases, the mire distortion is obvious on the video-keratograph (**a**). However, if it becomes too gross, it is difficult to reconstruct the topography (**b**), and some data points are either inaccurate or missing. In this situation, projection-based topography techniques are often more useful. This patient's more severely affected left eye is shown in Figs. 5.2, 5.3 and 5.5

Elevation Maps

Established disease is characterised by increased steepening of both anterior and posterior corneal surfaces, with the highest point being at the apex of the cone. Plotting the corneal shape as the difference from a best-fit sphere demonstrates the exaggerated prolate shape, with increased central steepening and peripheral

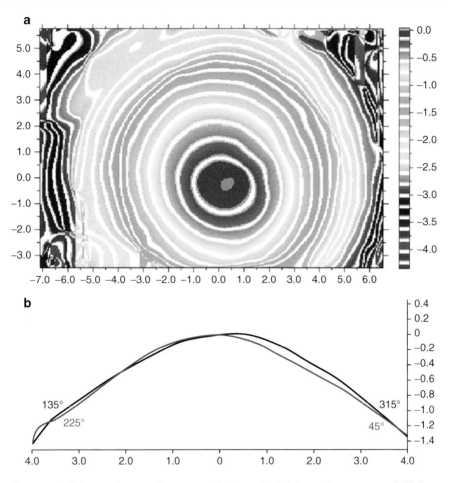

Fig. 10.4 Height maps in severe keratoconus. In this patient's left eye, the cone protruded infero-temporally. The images are obtained using moiré interference. (**a**) The apex of the cone is the highest point on the elevation map. The contours are closest together where the slope is steepest, on the inferotemporal side of the cone. (**b**) The cross-section in the 135° meridian (black) shows the inferotemporal protrusion and steepening, particularly compared to the perpendicular meridian (45°, red) which is relatively symmetric

flattening (Figs. 10.5a, b and 10.6). This can be useful for contact lens fitting in very irregular corneas, as the best-fit sphere can be set at the same radius of curvature as the posterior surface of a trial contact lens.

As a result of corneal thinning, the posterior surface often shows greater steepening than the anterior surface. In early keratoconus, this steepening on the posterior elevation map may be the first sign of keratoconus. Epithelial remodelling may mask steepening of the anterior corneal surface, due to epithelial thinning over the apex of the cone and thickening in an annulus surrounding it. This has been demonstrated using very-high-frequency ultrasound scanning (VHFUSS) [19–22].

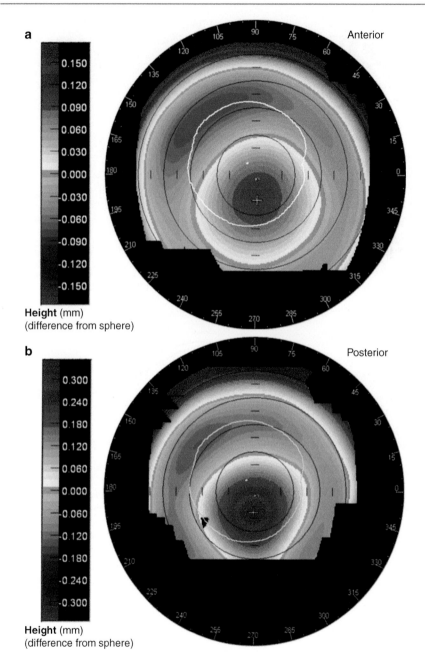

Fig. 10.5 Keratoconus measured by slit images. The topography of the anterior corneal surface of the right eye shows a prominent inferocentral cone (the reference sphere has a radius of curvature of 6.29 mm, which is equivalent to 53.7D). (**b**) The posterior surface shows a greater change in height from the periphery to the centre than the anterior surface (the reference sphere has a radius of curvature of 5.01 mm, which is equivalent to 67.4D. Note: the scale has double the interval of the map in part a). (**c**) Therefore, the pachymetric map shows that the central cornea is much thinner than normal (300 μ rather than 500–600 μ). (**d**) From the true height data, power can easily be calculated (Courtesy of Orbtek Incorporated, Salt Lake City, USA)

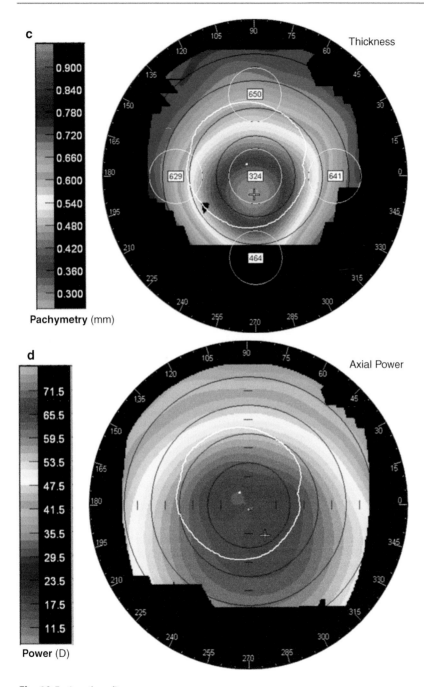

Fig. 10.5 (continued)

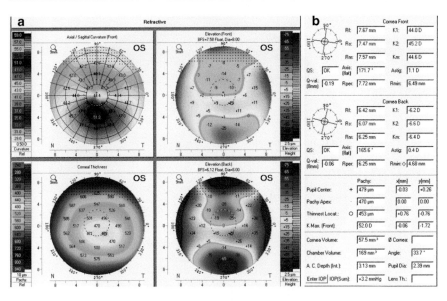

Fig. 10.6 (**a, b**) Subclinical keratoconus. The cornea appeared normal on biomicroscopic examination, but the topography revealed inferior steepening. This may represent a variation of normal or an early mild form of keratoconus / forme fruste keratoconus. A similar appearance is seen in Fig. 5.7

Pachymetric Maps

Corneal thinning can be another early sign of ectasia. In keratoconus it tends to be maximal at the apex of the cone paracentrally, whereas in pellucid marginal degeneration, this tends to be in the midperiphery inferiorly. In keratoglobus the thinning is more generalised, in all corneal meridians and out to the periphery. As well as being valuable in diagnosis, the corneal thickness can be helpful when planning surgery such as corneal collagen cross-linking or penetrating keratoplasty.

Slope Maps

The slope is zero at the apex of the cone and across the top of any focal protrusions such as proud nebulae (Fig. 5.5). These maps are particularly useful for very irregular corneas, in which local variations in height can be easily demonstrated.

Curvature and Power Maps

Colour-coded curvature or power maps of an eye with keratoconus show an asymmetric bow tie corresponding to the exaggerated prolate shape and irregular astigmatism of the corneal surface [15, 16] (Figs. 10.2b and 10.3b). In more severe cases, one of the bows of the bow tie may be absent.

Difference Maps

Direct comparison of two equivalent maps from different visits demonstrates change over time, whether it be due to progression or treatment. It is essential that the settings, as discussed earlier, are the same in order for the comparison to be valid. This is a valuable tool when monitoring patients for progression.

Keratoconus Detection Indices

Although the topography in moderate and severe cases of keratoconus is usually recognisable as such, the diagnosis can be more difficult in subtle cases or those with atypical topography. Uncertainty arises for two main reasons. Firstly, controversy still exists regarding the minimum topographic criteria for the diagnosis of keratoconus. Secondly, there is variation in the topographic patterns seen in this condition.

The interpretation of videokeratographs requires the examiner to have detailed knowledge and clinical experience of the subtle and complex patterns contained within them, in both normality and disease. In order to remove the subjectivity of the assessment and the need for experience, several authors have developed specific corneal indices and detection programmes designed to aid the topographic diagnosis of keratoconus [26–31]. In all cases, the maps and the indices should be interpreted in the light of the clinical findings. Some indices are specific to the software programmes of certain devices, but most devices incorporate some such indices and share certain principles in their design.

Indices are a way of quantifying the severity of keratoconus, which is valuable for tracking progress over time and for analysing grouped data in research studies. For example, in studies of the genetics of keratoconus, indices may provide quantitative information that can reflect the variable expression of the disease within family members. It can also quantify the differences in outcome between two treatments.

Indices are valuable in the detection of subclinical keratoconus, which is important for determining whether patients should be followed up to identify if they require cross-linking and whether they have an increased risk of complications if undergoing refractive surgery. Pattern recognition by an experienced observer can also be valuable in this role, although indices tend to be better than inexperienced observers.

Keratometry, Asymmetry and Regularity Indices

Quantitative descriptors were developed to quantify particular features of the corneal surface, which could then be correlated with the potential visual acuity [38, 39] (Chap. 5). For example, the surface asymmetry index (SAI) is a measure of the difference in corneal powers between points on the same ring 180° apart, over the entire corneal surface. The surface regularity index (SRI) is a measure of the local irregularity of the cornea within an area bounded by a virtual pupil 4.5 mm in diameter. It compares the power of each point with that of its immediate neighbours.

Although the asymmetry and the irregularity of the surface are often greater than normal in keratoconus, these indices are non-specific as they can also be elevated in other corneal diseases or following surgery. In addition, the SRI only uses data from the central cornea and may therefore miss important clues in the periphery. Several authors have developed indices which are specifically aimed at detecting keratoconus.

Inferior-Superior Value

The inferior-superior (I-S) value was designed to differentiate keratoconus from normal corneas [15]. It was defined as an average refractive power difference between five inferior points and five superior points 3 mm from the centre at 30° intervals. Although the I-S value is specifically seeking asymmetry between the superior and inferior hemispheres of the cornea, it may also be raised after penetrating keratoplasty or large incision cataract surgery. This shows the importance of knowing the history and biomicroscopic findings. In addition, the steepening in keratoconus is not always limited to the inferior periphery [16].

Difference in Central Power

The use of combinations of indices could improve their specificity in diagnosing keratoconus. The I-S value has been used in conjunction with the central corneal power and the difference in central power between fellow eyes [15]. However, central corneal power is a non-specific marker for keratoconus as some emmetropic eyes may have powers of 50.00D or more.

Keratoconus Predictability Index

Although single, relatively simple indices may be useful in distinguishing between keratoconus and normal corneas, more sophisticated methods are required to differentiate keratoconus from other clinical entities with similar topographic features. Accuracy can be improved by using a combination of indices. The keratoconus prediction index (KPI) is derived by inputting eight quantitative indices into an automated keratoconus detection algorithm [26] (Table 10.2). Each of the constituent indices quantifies a different aspect of the corneal surface in keratoconus. If, for a given cornea, the combined index is above the cut-off value, keratoconus is likely to be present. This method detects keratoconus with a sensitivity of 68%, specificity of 99% and accuracy of 90%.

The Belin-Ambrosio Enhanced Ectasia Display

The Belin-Ambrosio Enhanced Ectasia Display (BAD) combines elevation and pachymetric data and compares it to an "enhanced best-fit-sphere". This is calculated with a fixed optical zone of 8.0 mm, omitting the 4 mm around the elevated cone [32]. It performs regression analysis (including standard deviations (SD) from the mean) on changes in anterior and posterior elevation, corneal thickness at the thinnest point, thinnest point displacement and pachymetric progression. Using these values, it creates a new map, applying colours to represent variations from the mean. The Belin intuitive scale with 61 colours and a 2.5 μm step has been found to be the most reliable for displaying the elevation maps [22].

Table 10.2 The keratoconus predictability index (KPI) is derived by the discriminant analysis of eight corneal indices [434]

Keratoconus predictability index (KPI) derived by discriminant analysis of:		
Index	Description	Function
Simulated keratometry (max) (SimK1)	Power of the steepest meridian	Non-specific indicators
Simulated keratometry (min) (Sim K2)	Power of the flattest meridian	
Surface asymmetry index (SAI)	Difference in corneal power between points 180° apart	
Differential sector index (DSI)[a]	Difference in average power between sectors with greatest and least power	Detection of an area of significant localised steepening
Opposite sector index (OSI)[a]	Greatest difference in average power between any two opposite sectors	
Centre-surround index (CSI)[a]	Comparison of average power in central 3 mm zone and annulus from 3 to 6 mm	Differentiate between normal corneas, regular astigmatism, peripheral steepening keratoconus and central steepening keratoconus
Irregular astigmatism index (IAI)	Average power variation along each semimeridian	Detect corneal irregularity which can be associated with moderate and severe keratoconus
Analysed area (AA)	Ratio of the area of interpolated data to the area within the most peripheral mire	

To calculate the DSI and the OSI, the cornea was divided mathematically into eight pie-shaped sectors, each subtending 45°. This reference pattern was then rotated about the central axis, up to 45° in 32 incremental steps. The corneal sector with the greatest average area-corrected power was identified, and then the average area-corrected power was calculated for each of the remaining seven sectors

[a]The DSI, OSI and CSI use the concept of "area-corrected power". In videokeratographs peripheral data points provide information about a larger area of cornea than do central ones. Therefore each power was multiplied by the area of cornea from which it was derived. To calculate the average power for a region of the cornea, the sum of the area-corrected powers was divided by the area of that region

Automated Detection Programme for Subclinical Keratoconus

Incorporating more parameters into detection algorithms can enhance their reliability. An automated screening programme based on artificial intelligence has been developed utilising 56 parameters derived from topography, elevation maps, pachymetry and wavefront analysis. It uses the best-fit toric aspheric reference surface and has been shown to improve detection of subclinical keratoconus compared to the best-fit sphere (BFS) [35, 36]. The system is based on an automated decision tree algorithm that automatically selects variables that best discriminate the study population. This artificial intelligence system has the potential to improve the detection of mild ectatic corneas without requiring expertise in interpreting corneal imaging. It has been shown to detect subclinical keratoconus with 93.7% sensitivity and 97.2% specificity [36, 37].

Neural Networks
The accuracy of these indices can be further improved by using discriminant analysis embedded in an artificial intelligence mesh [26, 40]. Neural network models simulate some common aspects of the biological nervous system (Chap. 5). They contain facts and rules that enable them to make logic-based decisions. Information passing through a neural network is able to modify its components in a process simulating human "learning" in response to feedback. Therefore, with use and the input of human-determined diagnoses, the network is able to improve its recognition skills as it gains "experience". Using these techniques, the accuracy of detecting keratoconus improves to 96%.

Topographic Classification

Since the development of corneal topography, it has been possible to classify keratoconus on the basis of the appearance of colour-coded maps (Table 10.3). Several subsets have been identified based on the size, location and shape of the cone [16]. It is unknown to what degree these classifications have clinical importance. Further studies are required to investigate whether there are differences between subtypes in their aetiology, associations, progression and effect on visual performance.

Severity

The severity of keratoconus is related to the difference in power between the steepest and flattest portions of the cornea. The more severe cases are also associated with increasing surface irregularity and stromal thinning. The advent of corneal topography leads to the recognition of subclinical keratoconus, and the development of various indices has helped to distinguish these from normal corneas. Other systems have been developed to quantify the severity of established keratoconus.

Table 10.3 Classification of keratoconus.

Classification of keratoconus		
Severity	Site of cone	Shape of cone
Mild	Inferior	Typical/oval
Moderate	Central	Globus
Severe	Superior	Nipple

Amsler-Krumeich Classification

This is the oldest and most commonly used classification system. It is based on mean K readings on the anterior curvature sagittal map, the thickness at the thinnest location and the refractive error of the patient (see Table 10.4) [41, 42]. However, it does not utilise information which is now available due to technological advances in corneal imaging.

ABCD Classification

This new classification system combines information from the anterior (A) and posterior or back (B) radius of curvature (taken from the 3.0 mm zone centred in the thinnest point), the thinnest corneal (C) pachymetry and the distance (D) best-corrected vision. It adds a modifier for no scarring (−), for scarring that does not obscure iris details (+) or for scarring that does obscure iris details (++) (Table 10.5).

Table 10.4 The Amsler-Krumeich classification for grading keratoconus

Stage	Findings
1	Eccentric steepening
	Myopia, induced astigmatism, or both <5.00 D
	Mean central K readings <48 D
2	Myopia, induced astigmatism, or both from 5.00 to 8.00 D
	Mean central K readings <53.00 D
	Absence of scarring
	Corneal thickness >400 μ
3	Myopia, induced astigmatism, or both from 8.00 to 10.00 D
	Mean central K readings >53.00 D
	Absence of scarring
	Corneal thickness 300–400 μ
4	Refraction not measurable
	Mean central K readings >55.00 D
	Central corneal scarring
	Corneal thickness <200 μ

Table 10.5 ABCD grading system for classifying keratoconus

ABCD criteria	A ARC (3 mm zone)	B PRC (3 mm zone)	C Thinnest pachy (μm)	D BDVA	Scarring
Stage 0	>7.25 mm (<46.5D)	>5.90 mm (<57.25D)	>490	≥20/20	−
Stage 1	>7.05 mm (<48.0D)	>5.70 mm (<59.25D)	>450	>20/20	−,+,++
Stage 2	>6.35 mm (<53.0D)	>5.15 mm (<65.5D)	>400	<20/40	−,+,++
Stage 3	>6.15 mm (<55.0D)	>4.95 mm (<68.5D)	>300	<20/100	−,+,++
Stage 4	<6.15 mm (>55.0D)	<4.95 mm (>68.5D)	≤300	<20/400	−,+,++

It utilises the central 3 mm zone centred on the thinnest point because this area better represents the ectatic region than a single point parameter such as Kmax or maximal elevation [43].

Location

The cone is most commonly positioned either inferiorly or inferocentrally. Other much rarer presentations include central (Fig. 10.7) and superior (Fig. 10.8). However, one study suggests that the principal steepening was above the horizontal meridian in as many as 17% of corneas [50, 51], although it is less frequently so in most clinical practice.

Shape

Most cones have an oval shape on topography usually involving one or two quadrants (Fig. 10.2b). Outside these affected areas, the topography may have a relatively "normal" appearance. Nipple-shaped and globus cones are much less

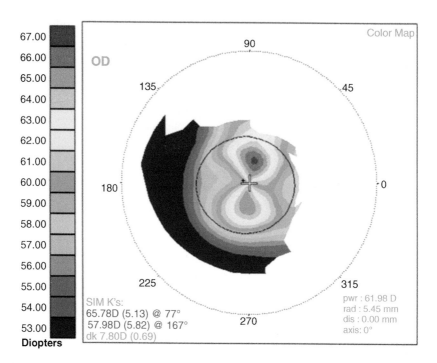

Fig. 10.7 Central keratoconus. In this patient with the classic biomicroscopic signs of keratoconus, the central cornea is usually steep. The bow tie is relatively symmetric and is contained almost entirely within the 4 mm optical zone

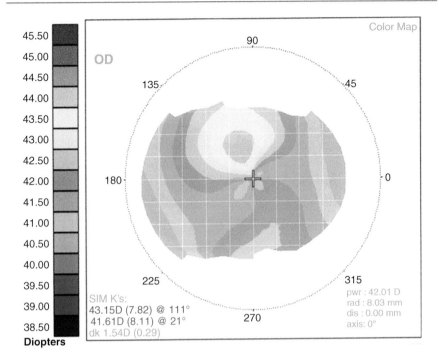

Fig. 10.8 Superior keratoconus. The irregular asymmetric bow tie has its steepest portion in the superior cornea

common. Nipple-shaped cones are much more localised (≤5 mm in diameter) and are usually round, relatively central and completely surrounded by relatively flat "normal" cornea (Figs. 10.9 and 10.10). In the globus variety, the cone is extensive and involves up to three-quarters of the corneal surface. This probably represents a clinical overlap with keratoglobus [13, 14, 25].

Information regarding the shape and extent of the cone can be of importance for optimal contact lens fitting, especially for the nipple and globus varieties when aspheric shapes are preferable.

Differential Diagnosis

Significant paracentral corneal steepening is not unique to keratoconus (Table 10.1). Before the diagnosis is confirmed, other conditions causing a similar appearance should be excluded.

Artefact
Eccentric fixation by the patient or decentration of the topography equipment can produce maps resembling keratoconus when the cornea is in fact normal [52, 53]

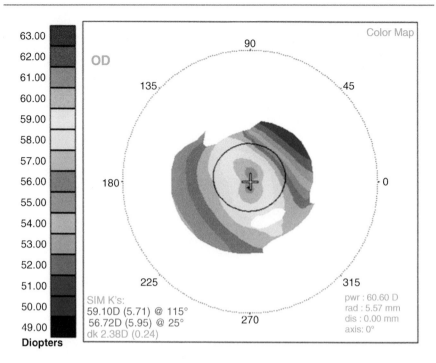

Fig. 10.9 Nipple keratoconus. The central cornea is almost spherical and is much steeper than the surrounding peripheral cornea

(Fig. 6.7). If there is any doubt or the patient appears to have subclinical keratoconus, the examination should be performed again with particular attention given to fixation and alignment.

Contact Lens-Induced Corneal Warpage
Inferior corneal steepening can result from corneal warpage due to superiorly decentred rigid contact lenses [27] (Fig. 7.8). This may persist for many weeks after lens removal.

Corneal Disease
Keratoconus forms part of the spectrum of corneal ectatic diseases which also includes keratoglobus and pellucid marginal degeneration [54] (Fig. 9.6).

Corneal Surgery
Localised corneal steepening may result from penetrating keratoplasty, epikeratophakia, hyperopic photorefractive keratectomy and other refractive procedures (Fig. 14.4). However, the aetiology should be apparent from the history and biomicroscopic examination.

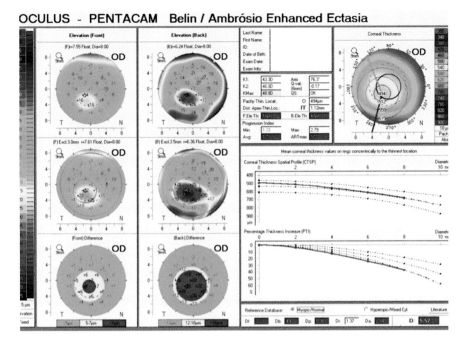

Fig. 10.10 Shows the display for the BAD in a patient with KCN. The top two elevation maps are the regular elevation maps relative to the standard BFS with the front and back surfaces on the left and right respectively. The radius of the BFS and diameter of the zone used are at the top of each picture. In the middle pictures are the enhanced or exclusion maps which reference the enhanced BAD BFS. A red circle marks its location. The bottom pictures show the difference between the standard elevation and enhanced or exclusion maps. Green represents normal cornea with a change of less than 5 μm on the anterior surface and 12 μm on the posterior surface of the cornea; yellow indicates suspicious cornea (at least 1.6 SD from the mean) with a change of between 5–12 μm for the anterior surface and 12–16 μm for the posterior surface. A value of +15 at the thinnest point warrants suspicion as it occurs in less than 1% of normal corneas.[45] Red indicates an abnormal cornea (at least 2.6 SD from the mean) with a change greater than 7 μm anteriorly and greater than 16 posteriorly. In normal eyes, an average elevation value at the thinnest point is 3.6 ± 4.7 μm with a cut off for keratoconus at 14 μm [33, 34]

Contact Lens Fitting

Computerised videokeratoscopy / scheimpflug imaging can be of great value in the contact lens management of keratoconus both in early and severe cases [55] (Chap. 7). Traditionally keratometry has been used to fit lenses in such eyes. However, keratometry readings, which only obtain data from four points within the central 3.0 mm of the cornea, can be inaccurate and may even be misleading in eyes with keratoconus.

Subtraction of height data from a best-fit sphere demonstrates the mismatch in shape between the anterior surface of the cornea and the posterior surface of a contact lens. This is particularly helpful in cases with corneal irregularities such as proud nebulae.

Penetrating Keratoplasty

Serial topography after penetrating keratoplasty for keratoconus has revealed large configurational changes in the 1st month after surgery, which can then remain relatively stable until suture removal [56]. Topographic analysis has been more effectively used than keratometry to identify the steep meridian after keratoplasty because it examines a large rea of cornea rather than the central 3 mm. It has been used to direct selective suture removal to reduce astigmatism after surgery and enhance visual performance (Chap. 11). However, removal of tight sutures and not those of normal tension can just result in a change in the axis of the astigmatism because the region of the removed suture is then flatter than the areas on either side where the sutures remain.

Topography is also more accurate for planning subsequent astigmatic keratotomy and laser corneal refractive procedures (Chap. 13).

In some eyes, astigmatism may increase gradually many years after surgery. It has been thought that this represents either recurrence of the disease in the graft [57] or the presence of undiagnosed keratoconus in the donor material [58]. The use of topography may elucidate the true incidence of recurrent disease. In addition, topographic analysis may provide a better understanding of the effects of surgical variables such as graft size and decentration on the optical results after penetrating keratoplasty [59].

References

*References Particularly Worth Reading

1. Rabinowitz YS, Maumenee IH, Lundergan MK. Molecular genetic analysis in autosomal dominant keratoconus. Cornea. 1992;11:302–8.
2. Rabinowitz YS, Garbus J, McDonnell PJ. Computer-assisted corneal topography in family members of patients with keratoconus. Arch Ophthalmol. 1990;108:365–71.
3. Gonzalez V, McDonnell PJ. Computer-assisted corneal topography in parents of patients with keratoconus. Arch Ophthalmol. 1992;110:1412–4.
4. *Rabinowitz YS, Nesburn AB, McDonnell PJ. Videokeratography of the fellow eye in unilateral keratoconus. Ophthalmology. 1993;100:181–186.
5. Behrens-Baumann W. Detection of keratoconus before refractive surgery [letter]. Ophthalmology. 1994;101:794–5.
6. Hustead JD. Detection of keratoconus before keratorefractive surgery [letter]. Ophthalmology. 1993;100:975.
7. *Holland DR, Maeda N, Hannush SB, Riveroll LH, Green MT, Klyce SD, Wilson SE. Unilateral keratoconus. Ophthalmology. 1997;104:1409–1413.

8. Eran P, Almogit A, David Z, et al. The D144E substitution in the VSX1 gene: a non-pathogenic variant or a disease causing mutation? Ophthalmic Genet. 2008;29:53–9.

9. Sherwin T, Brookes NH, Loh IP, et al. Cellular incursion into Bowman's membrane in the peripheral cone of the keratoconic cornea. Exp Eye Res. 2002;74(4):473–82.

10. Mas-Tur V, MacGregor C, Jayaswal R, et al. A review of keratoconus: diagnosis, pathophysiology and genetics. Surv Ophthalmol. 2017;62(6):770–83.

11. Tuft SJ, Moodaley LC, Gregory WM, Davison CR, Buckley RJ. Prognostic factors for the progression of keratoconus. Ophthalmology. 1994;101:439–47.

12. Karolak JA, Kulinska K, Nowak DM, et al. Sequence variants in COL4A1 and COL4A2 genes in Ecuadorian families with keratoconus. Mol Vis. 2011;17:827–43.

13. Mintz-Hittner HA, Semina EV, Frishman LJ, et al. VSX1 (RINX) mutation with craniofacial anomalies, empty sella, corneal endothelial changes and abnormal retinal and auditory bipolar cells. Ophthalmology. 2004;111:828–36.

14. Godefrooij DA, Ardine de Wit G, Uiterwaal CS, et al. Age-specific incidence and prevalence of keratoconus: a nationwide registration study. Am J Ophthalmol. 2017;175:169–72.

15. *Rabinowitz YS, McDonnell PJ. Computer-assisted corneal topography in keratoconus. Refract Corneal Surg. 1989;5:400–408.

16. *Wilson SE, Lin DTC, Klyce SD. Corneal topography of keratoconus. Cornea. 1991;10:2–8.

17. de Cunha DA, Woodward EG. Measurement of corneal topography in keratoconus. Ophthal Physiol Opt. 1993;13:377–82.

18. Corbett MC, O'Brart DPS, Stultiens BAT, Jongsma FHM, Marshall J. Corneal topography using a new moiré image-based system. Eur J Implant Ref Surg. 1995;7:353–70.

19. Mok JW, Baek SJ, Joo CK, et al. VSX1 gene variants are associated with keratoconus in unrelated Korean patients. J Hum Genet. 2008;53:842–9.

20. Reinstein DZ, Archer TJ, Gobbe M. Corneal epithelial thickness profile in the diagnosis of keratoconus. J Refract Surg. 2009;25(7):604–10.

21. Maguire LJ, Bourne MW. Corneal topography of early keratoconus (reply). Am J Ophthalmol. 1989;108:747–8.

22. Belin MW, Khachikian SS. An introduction to understanding elevation based topography: how elevation data are displayed – a review. Clin Exp Ophthalmol. 2009;37:14–29.

23. Li X, Bykhovskaya Y, Canedo AL, et al. Genetic association of COL5A1 variants in keratoconus patients suggests a complex connection between corneal thinning and keratoconus. IOVS. 2013;54(4):2696–704.

24. Sharma A, Tovey JC, Ghosh A, et al. AAV serotype influences gene transfer in corneal stroma in vivo. Exp Eye Res. 2010;3:440–8.

25. Manuolio TA. Genome-wide association studies and assessment of the risk of disease. N Engl J Med. 2010;2:166–76.

26. *Madea N, Klyce SD, Smolek MK, Thompson HW. Automated keratoconus screening with corneal topography analysis. Invest Ophthalmol Vis Sci. 1994;35:2749–2757.

27. Smolek MK, Klyce SD, Maeda N. Keratoconus and contact lens-induced corneal warpage analysis using the keratomorphic diagram. Invest Ophthalmol Vis Sci. 1994;35:4192–203.

28. Maeda N, Klyce SD, Smolek MK. Comparison of methods for detecting keratoconus using videokeratoscopy. Arch Ophthalmol. 1995;113:870–4.

29. Goren MB. Comparison of methods for detecting keratoconus using videokeratography [letter]. Arch Ophthalmol. 1996;114:631.

30. Klyce SD, Smolek MK, Maeda N. Comparison of methods for detecting keratoconus using videokeratography [reply]. Arch Ophthalmol. 1996;114:631–2.

31. *Smolek MK, Klyce SD. Current keratoconus detection methods compared with a neural network approach. Invest Ophthalmol Vis Sci. 1997;38:2290–2299.

32. Ambrosio R Jr, Alonson RS, Luz A, et al. Corneal thickness spatial profile and corneal volume distribution: tomographic indices to detect keratoconus. J Cat Refract Surg. 2006;32(11):1851–9.

33. Abad JC, Rubinfeld RS, Del Valle M, et al. Vertical D: a novel topographic pattern in some keratoconus suspects. Ophthalmology. 2007;114(5):1020–6.

34. Khachikian SS, Belin MW. Posterior elevation in keratoconus. Ophthalmology. 2009;116(4):816e1.
35. Arce C. Qualitative and quantitative analysis of aspheric symmetry and asymmetry on corneal surfaces. ASCRS (American Society of Cataract and Refractive Surgeons) Conference: Boston; 2010.
36. Smadja D, Touboul D, Cohen A, et al. Detection of subclinical keratoconus using an automated decision tree classification. Am J Ophthalmol. 2013;156(2):237–246e1.
37. Maeda N, Klyce SD, Smolek MK, et al. Automated keratoconus screening with corneal topography analysis. IOVS. 1994;35(6):2749–57.
38. Dingeldein SA, Klyce SD, Wilson SE. Quantitative descriptors of corneal shape derived from the computer-assisted analysis of photokeratographs. Refract Corneal Surg. 1989;5:372–8.
39. Wilson SE, Klyce SD. Quantitative descriptors of corneal topography. A clinical study. Arch Ophthalmol. 1991;109:349–53.
40. Maeda M, Klyce SD, Smolek MK. Neural network classification of corneal topography. Invest Ophthalmol Vis Sci. 1995;36:1327–35.
41. Amsler M. Le keratocone fruste au javal. Ophthalmologica. 1938;96:77–83.
42. Amsler M. Keratocone classique et keratocone fruste, arguments unitaire. Ophthalmologica. 1946;111:96–101.
43. Belin MW, Duncan J, Ambrosio R Jr, et al. A new tomographic method of grading keratoconus: the ABCD Grading system. Int J Kerat Ect Cor Dis. 2015;4(3):85–93.
44. *Wilson SE, Klyce SD. Screening for corneal topographic abnormalities before refractive surgery. Ophthalmology. 1994;101:147–152.
45. Nesburn AB, Bahri S, Salz J, Rabinowitz YS, Maguen E, Hofbauer J, Belin M, Macy JI. Keratoconus detected by videokeratography in candidates for photorefractive keratectomy. J Refract Surg. 1995;11:194–201.
46. Bowman CB, Thompson KP, Stulting RD. Refractive keratotomy in keratoconus suspects. J Refract Surg. 1995;11:202–6.
47. Doyle SJ, Hynes E, Naroo S, Shah S. PRK in patients with a keratoconic topography picture. The concept of a physiological 'displaced apex syndrome'. Br J Ophthalmol. 1996;80:25–8.
48. Colin J, Cochener B, Bobo C, Malet F, Gallinaro C, Le Floch G. Myopic photorefractive keratectomy in eyes with atypical inferior corneal steepening. J Cat Refract Surg. 1996;22:1423–6.
49. O'Brart DPS, Saunders DC, Corbett MC, Rosen ES. The corneal topography of keratoconus. Eur J Implant Ref Surg. 1995;7(1):20–30.
50. Eiferman RA, Lane L, Law M, Fields Y. Superior keratoconus [letter]. Refract Corneal Surg. 1993;9:394–5.
51. *McMahon TT, Robin JB, Scarpulla KM, Putz JL. The spectrum of corneal topography found in keratoconus. CLAO J. 1991;17:198–204.
52. *Hubbe RE, Foulks GN. The effect of poor fixation on computer-assisted topographic corneal analysis. Ophthalmology. 1994;101:1745–1748.
53. Silverman CM. Misalignment of videokeratoscope produces pseudo-keratoconus suspect. J Cat Refract Surg. 1994;10:468.
54. *Karabatsas CH, Cook SD. Topographic analysis in pellucid marginal degeneration and keratoglobus. Eye. 1996;10:451–455.
55. *Rabinowitz YS, Garbus JJ, Garbus C, McDonnell PJ. Contact lens selection for keratoconus using a computer assisted videokeratoscope. CLAO J. 1991;17:88–93.
56. Khong AM, Mannis MJ, Plotnik RD, Johnson CA. Computerised topographic analysis of the healing graft after penetrating keratoplasty for keratoconus. Am J Ophthalmol. 1993;115:209–15.
57. Kremer I, Eagle RC, Rapuano CJ, Laibson PR. Histological evidence of recurrent keratoconus seven years after keratoplasty. Am J Ophthalmol. 1995;199:511–2.
58. Bechrakis N, Blom ML, Stark WJ, Green WR. Recurrent keratoconus. Cornea. 1994;13:73–7.
59. Serdarevic ON, Renard GJ, Pouliquen Y. Penetrating keratoplasty for keratoconus: role of videokeratoscopy and trephine sizing. J Cataract Refract Surg. 1996;22:1165–74.

Part IV

Corneal Surgery

Keratoplasty

11

Any form of ocular surgery has the potential to alter the surface topography of the cornea. In some cases such as refractive and certain corneal procedures, this is the desired effect (Chaps. 12, 13 and 14), but in other cases, the changes induced may lead to a reduction in postoperative visual performance (Chaps. 11, 12, 15). This section describes how a variety of ocular procedures can influence corneal topography.

All surgical operations consist of a series of planned manoeuvres and traumatic events, each of which can act through one or more mechanisms to influence corneal shape [1–3]. The effect of each mechanism in individual patients is modified by the preoperative and postoperative environment (Table 11.1). In this chapter, the basic principles underlying these mechanisms are described, using keratoplasty as an example of a fundamental corneal procedure.

In patients undergoing keratoplasty, corneal topography is valuable preoperatively to assess corneal astigmatism and postoperatively to guide suture removal or subsequent refractive surgery. In addition, analysis of the information provided has been used to improve surgery and optimise visual outcome. Intraoperative keratoscopy is valuable for modifying corneal shape during surgery, either by guiding the length and depth of incisions or through the adjustment of the tension of corneal sutures.

Mechanisms

Corneal surgery can induce topographic changes both directly, at the site of the surgical trauma, and indirectly at distant sites as a result of "coupling". Direct effects include local changes to the corneal epithelium, stroma or overlying tear fluid (Chap. 8). Indirect effects occur when corneal incisions are deep enough, or forces are great enough, to disrupt the mechanical integrity of the cornea by destabilising the shape and arrangement of collagen fibres in the corneal stromal lamellae

© Springer Nature Switzerland AG 2019   171
M. Corbett et al., *Corneal Topography*,
https://doi.org/10.1007/978-3-030-10696-6_11

Table 11.1 Factors affecting the topographic outcome of corneal surgery

Factors affecting topographic outcome of corneal surgery	
Preoperative	Corneal disease
	Pre-existing astigmatism
Intraoperative	Incision
	Location
	Length
	Depth
	Architecture
	Wound closure
	Alignment
	Suture bites – length, depth and tension
	Suture orientation
	Suture material
Postoperative	Suture adjustment
	Wound healing
	Therapeutic agents
	Complications
	Infection
	Inflammation
	Vascularisation

(Chap. 9). Following a surgical procedure, several mechanisms may be effective simultaneously, and their interaction can generate complex topographic patterns.

In each case, the primary topographic change can be classified as corneal steepening, corneal flattening or irregular astigmatism (Fig. 11.1).

Corneal Steepening

Corneal steepening is most commonly the result of a tight suture in the corneal periphery (Fig. 11.1a). Tissue compression within the suture bite depresses the limbal cornea towards the centre of the globe, thereby increasing the curvature of the central cornea [1, 2]. This is associated with a small area of flattening immediately within the area of the suture and a secondary flattening in the meridian perpendicular to the suture, as a result of coupling (Fig. 11.2).

Localised corneal steepening may result from vertical wound misalignment in which the central edge under-rides the peripheral edge. Other local causes include oedema of the wound margin, proud scar tissue or cautery causing tissue contraction [4] (Fig. 11.1b).

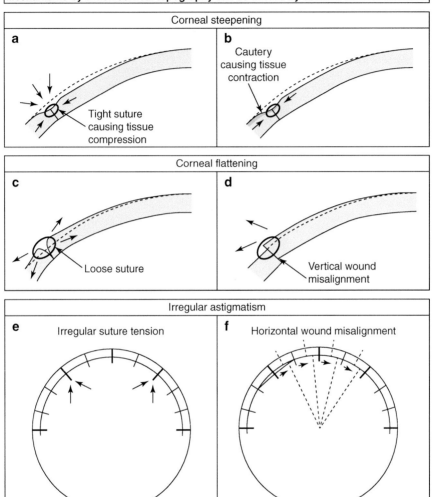

Fig. 11.1 Surgically induced astigmatism. Sutured corneal incisions such as those made during corneal graft surgery or extracapsular cataract extraction can alter corneal topography by wound compression, gape or misalignment. (**a–d**) are cross sections through the cornea at the site of the incision. (Arrows = direction of the forces exerted; dashed lines = original position of the corneal surface.) In (**e**) and (**f**), the cornea is viewed from anteriorly (Arrows indicate tight sutures in (**e**) and the wound misalignment in (**f**); dashed lines would have been continuous prior to surgery in (**f**))

Fig. 11.2 Regular corneal
graft astigmatism (steep).
Regular astigmatism due to
particularly tight sutures at
0° and 180°. This has the
appearance of a horizontal
red bow tie because the
cornea is prolate (steeper
in the centre than the
periphery). Coupling has
resulted in flattening of the
perpendicular meridian

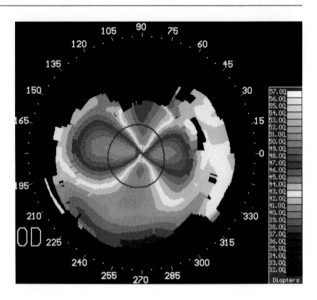

Corneal Flattening

Corneal flattening is most commonly due to wound gape [1]. This is sometimes seen
to a minor extent in small unsutured wounds but more commonly in larger wounds
with inadequate support or closure (Fig. 10.1c). At the time of surgery, sutures may
be too few in number or tied too loosely. Sutures placed too superficially may result
in posterior wound gape, which has a similar topographic appearance [5].
Postoperatively, sutures may become loose as a result of cheese-wiring, knot-
slippage, suture-related inflammation, degradation of absorbable sutures or prema-
ture removal. Similarly, any process that delays or impairs wound healing such as
infection or the use of intensive or prolonged postoperative topical corticosteroid
regimens can be associated with wound gape [6].

Wound gape increases the circumference of the globe in the meridian perpendicular to the line of the incision, thereby flattening the incisional meridian (Figs. 11.3,
12.2 and 12.3). If the wound edges are in poor apposition and the gaping area is filled
by fibrovascular scar tissue, this may later stretch leading to increased corneal flattening. Coupling frequently results in steepening of the perpendicular meridian.

Vertical misalignment of the wound with the central edge over-riding the peripheral edge also produces wound-related corneal flattening (Fig. 11.1d). Other localised causes include stromal compression, tissue destruction, subepithelial fibrosis
[7] or disruption of the air-tear fluid-epithelium interface.

Irregular Astigmatism

Astigmatism is most likely to be regular if due to either a single or a uniform
structural defect. This is usually relatively easy to correct either optically or

Fig. 11.3 Regular corneal graft astigmatism (flat). Astigmatism due to particularly loose sutures at 120° and 285°. This has the appearance of a vertical blue bow tie because the cornea is oblate (flatter in the centre than the periphery). This has arisen from the suturing being rather loose overall. Coupling has resulted in steepening of the perpendicular meridian

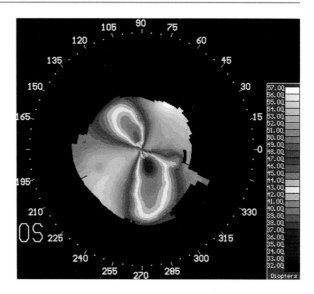

Fig. 11.4 Asymmetrical corneal graft astigmatism. Keratometry and refraction agreed that the steep axis was at 50°. However, corneal topography revealed the 230° semimeridian was much steeper than the 50° semimeridian. Sutures would need to be removed from 90° arc inferiorly but only a 20° arc superiorly

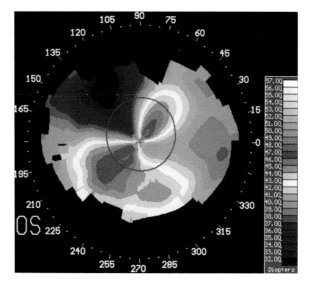

surgically. However, more complex anatomical changes can result in irregular astigmatism, which produces greater visual dysfunction and is more difficult to correct [8, 9]. Bi-oblique astigmatism (non-perpendicular axes) may occur if nonadjacent sutures are overtightened (Fig. 11.1e). A torsional effect results from a horizontal misalignment of the wound, whether due to a mismatching of its edges or non-radial suture bites (Fig. 11.1f). Areas of both wound gape and compression occur, resulting in complex and irregular topographic patterns (Figs. 11.4, 11.5 and 11.6).

Fig. 11.5 Irregular corneal graft astigmatism. The instantaneous axes show that the steep meridians are at an angle to each other (oblique astigmatism) (**a**). Removal of the tight sutures thus identified reduced the magnitude of the astigmatism and rendered it regular (**b**) and amenable to optical correction

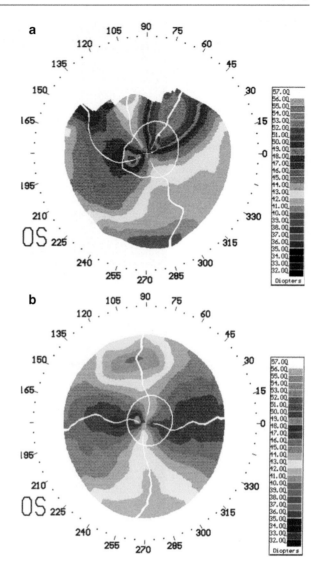

Topography After Keratoplasty

Corneal transplantation may involve either full-thickness (penetrating) or partial-thickness (lamellar) keratoplasty. In either technique, procedures involving the majority of the anterior layers of the cornea (penetrating, deep anterior lamellar or tectonic) can generate substantial changes in the corneal topography, whereas those involving thin or posterior layers (endothelial keratoplasty) have little effect.

Penetrating keratoplasty is the type of corneal transplantation that has been studied most. The procedure involves a 360° incision and replacement of the whole of

Fig. 11.6 Steep-flat
corneal graft astigmatism.
In this form or irregular
astigmatism, the cornea is
steeper on one side and
becomes progressively
flatter towards the other
side

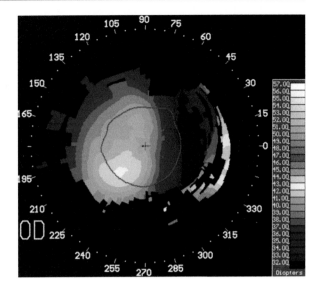

the central cornea, so the resulting topographic appearances are varied and may be
highly irregular and non-physiological. The videokeratoscopic patterns have been
described using both simple [10] and more complicated [11] classifications. Both
systems utilise the shape of the corneal profile and the presence of asymmetry and
irregularity.

Classification

The corneal profile is classified as prolate if the centre is steeper than the periphery,
oblate if the centre is flatter than the periphery or mixed (Figs. 11.2 and 11.3).
Asymmetry is present if the ends of the bow tie are significantly different sizes
(Fig. 11.4) and irregularity if they are at an angle to one another (Fig. 11.5). Other
irregular patterns are classified according to their appearance (Fig. 11.6, Table 11.2).

After penetrating keratoplasty, the ends of a bow tie are frequently wedge-
shaped, with straight edges (Fig. 11.7), rather than the "figure-of-eight" configuration with rounded ends seen in normal corneas. This occurs because the donor
button, once removed from the surrounding cornea, tends to be spherical in cross
section, rather than prolate, and the shape has less continuity with that of the surrounding host cornea.

Incidence

The reported incidence of topographic patterns varies between studies (Table 11.3).
This is because small variations in surgical technique can have markedly different
effects on corneal topography. With modern advances in eye banking and

Table 11.2 Classification of topographic patterns occurring after penetrating keratoplasty [913]

Classification of topography after keratoplasty	
Pattern	Description
Non-astigmatic	Round
Regular astigmatism	Angle between axis of two halves of bow tie <20°
Oval	Ratio shortest: longest diameter <2/3
Prolate	Steeper centrally than peripherally (red bow tie)
Symmetric bow tie	Ratio small bow: large bow >2/3, or difference < 1D
Prolate	Steeper centrally than peripherally (red bow tie)
Asymmetric bow tie	Ratio small bow: large bow <2/3, or difference >1D
Oblate	Flatter centrally than peripherally (blue bow tie)
Symmetric bow tie	Ratio small bow: large bow >2/3, or difference < 1D
Oblate	Flatter centrally than peripherally (blue bow tie)
Asymmetric bow tie	Ratio small bow: large bow <2/3, or difference >1D
Irregular astigmatism	
Mixed	Steep/flat pattern with bow tie
Prolate	Steeper centrally than peripherally (red bow tie)
Irregular	Angle between axis of two halves of bow tie >20°
Oblate	Steeper centrally than peripherally (blue bow tie)
Irregular	Angle between axis of two halves of bow tie >20°
Horseshoe pattern	Partial annulus of increased corneal power at graft-host interface
Triple pattern	Three distinct areas of radial steepening
Steep/flat pattern	Steeper on one side, becoming progressively flatter towards the other side
Localised steep pattern	Eccentric area of localised steepness, <25% of corneal diameter
Unclassified	

Fig. 11.7 Truncated bow tie pattern. After penetrating keratoplasty, the ends of the bow tie are frequently wedge-shaped with straight edges because the donor button tends to be more spherical than prolate, once removed from the scleral ring

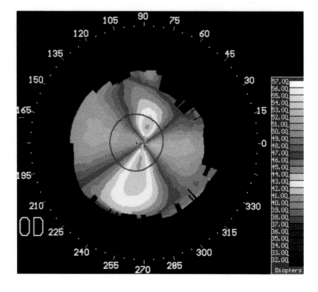

Table 11.3 Incidence of the various topographic patterns at least 1 year after penetrating kerato-plasty [913, 781]

Karabatsas et al. [11] (n = 85)			Tripoli et al. [10] (n = 45)	
Non-astigmatic	5%	5%		
Regular astigmatism	24%			
Oval		4%		
Prolate Symmetric bow tie		0%	Prolate	31%
Prolate Asymmetric bow tie		7%		
Oblate Symmetric bow tie		7%	Oblate	31%
Oblate Asymmetric bow tie		6%		
Irregular astigmatism	72%			
Mixed		8%	Mixed	18%
Prolate Irregular		6%	Asymmetric	9%
Oblate Irregular		5%		
Horseshoe pattern		4%		
Triple pattern		4%		
Steep/flat pattern		13%	Steep/flat	13%
Localised steep pattern		19%		
Unclassified		14%		

microsurgical techniques, optically clear grafts can be obtained in a high percentage of cases. However, postoperative astigmatism is still a significant factor that often limits visual rehabilitation [12–16]. It has been estimated that approximately 10% of penetrating keratoplasties have more than 5.00DC of keratometric astigmatism [17], and in keratoconic eyes, this may be as high as 27% [18].

Recent data from the National Health Service Blood and Ocular Tissue Advisory Group has shown stable visual outcomes 2–5 years following penetrating or endothelial keratoplasty [19]. The majority of keratoconus patients with a penetrating keratoplasty (PK) or deep anterior lamellar keratoplasty maintained their visual acuity (651/868; 75%), whilst 15% (133/868) improved and 10% (84/868) deteriorated. Similarly, most patients with Fuchs endothelial dystrophy (FED) who received a PK maintained their vision (395/569; 70%), whilst 18% (105/569) improved and 12% (68/569) deteriorated.

Modifying Factors

Although the topographic outcome of surgery is highly dependent upon surgical technique, it is also modified by preoperative and postoperative factors

Table 11.4 Factors affecting the topographic outcome of penetrating keratoplasty

Factors affecting topographic outcome of penetrating keratoplasty	
Preoperative	Corneal disease in recipient
	Corneal thickness
	Previous surgery
	Pre-existing astigmatism in donor or recipient cornea
Intraoperative	Trephination of donor and recipient
	Relative sizes
	Precision (e.g. centring, verticality, ledges)
	Alignment of the donor cornea in the recipient
	Suture technique
	Tension
	Length
	Depth
	Orientation
Postoperative	Suture adjustment
	Wound healing or dehiscence
	Graft rejection
	Recurrence of original pathology
	Complications
	Infection
	Inflammation
	Vascularisation
	Trauma

(Table 11.4). There are numerous studies within the literature based on refractive and keratometric data which attempt to examine the relative importance of each.

The development of corneal topography has provided a powerful investigative tool with which such factors can be examined in greater detail. For example, videokeratoscopy has been used to investigate diurnal variation in corneal shape after keratoplasty [20] and the rate and pattern of postoperative stabilisation in cases of keratoconus [21]. Further topographic studies should both improve our understanding of the pathogenesis of astigmatism after keratoplasty and allow the development of surgical strategies to minimise and correct it.

Preoperative Factors

The ease and the outcome of surgery are partially determined by the state of the cornea preoperatively. Corneal topography can help in the selection of the appropriate size of graft. In cases such as keratoconus, the area of cornea affected by irregular astigmatism can be identified and encompassed by a sufficiently large trephine. Slit photography systems (Chap. 3) can measure corneal pachymetry to identify thin areas to be avoided by the graft-host junction. In addition, knowledge of the uniformity of corneal thickness under the trephine can help the surgeon avoid creating irregularities of the graft-host interface.

Intraoperative Factors

For all types of anterior segment surgery, the factors with greatest influence on postoperative corneal topography are the incision and its closure.

Incisions

The characteristics of the incisions selected for a particular procedure will depend upon whether it is intended to alter the topography of the cornea. Refractive procedures aim to maximise the effect of an incision on the topography, whereas non-refractive procedures will aim to minimise these effects.

Incision Location
The closer a wound is made to the corneal centre, the greater its effect on the corneal topography [22]. Induced astigmatism is less for larger corneal grafts than for small ones and for cataract incisions made in the sclera or limbus than those in the cornea [23–25].

Incision Length
Larger incisions tend to induce greater changes in topography than short ones. This has been clearly demonstrated by small incision cataract surgery in which 2 mm wounds are associated with much less astigmatism than procedures performed through 12–13 mm wounds and less than even those performed through 5 mm incisions [4, 8, 24, 26–32]. Penetrating keratoplasty represents an extreme situation in which the incision involves 360° of the corneal circumference, as opposed to 30–40° or 120° in cataract surgery. With increasing incision length, there is a correspondingly greater risk that the astigmatism induced will be irregular.

Incision Depth
Increasing depth of incision is also associated with greater topographic changes. The use of lamellar keratoplasty reduces the risk of astigmatism compared to a full-thickness procedure. Similarly with radial keratotomy, if the refractive effect of the initial procedure is insufficient, augmentation may be performed by increasing the depth of the original incisions.

Incision Architecture
Over recent years, there have been attempts to minimise the corneal astigmatism induced during ocular surgery by altering the cross-sectional profile of wounds [24, 33, 34]. Many different profiles have been investigated, including vertical, those bevelled anteriorly or posteriorly and two-, three- or four-stepped incisions.

In corneal graft surgery, the wound margins should be as vertical as possible without any unintended notches or ledges, so that the donor closely opposes the host. The buttons are usually centred on the corneal landmarks rather than the site of disease in order to minimise astigmatism. Most surgeons oversize the diameter of the donor button by 0.25 mm relative to the host to compensate for elastic contraction of the corneal tissue and to avoid leaks. Oversizing by 0.5 mm may result in corneal steepening, whilst the use of the same sized trephine for both donor and host may produce corneal flattening.

For cataract surgery incisions, some investigators have attributed importance to the horizontal component of the wound profile. It has been postulated that by creating a tunnel or flap, the increased surface area for healing will result in greater wound stability and will in turn lessen any postoperative changes in topography.

Wound Closure

Non-astigmatic wound closure requires that the wound margins should be accurately aligned and held securely in position by sutures of the appropriate tension.

Alignment

During wound closure, appropriate alignment of the margins of the incision is essential. Vertical misalignment causes regular local steepening or flattening, whilst horizontal misalignment is associated with irregular astigmatism (Fig. 11.1).

In large-incision cataract surgery, the ends of the incision are tethered, and the two margins of the wound should match. Therefore, alignment just requires that the tissues should be returned to their original position. For large incisions, some surgeons insert preplaced sutures before making the corneal incision full-thickness, to ensure accurate alignment of the wound edges [9].

However, in keratoplasty, the two wound margins may match less well, particularly if there is irregular astigmatism in the host or corneal disease affecting the graft-host junction. If the tissue on either side of the wound is of different thicknesses, care must be taken that the suture bites are of equal depth. An additional problem in keratoplasty is that the donor tissue is freely mobile, and therefore the positioning of the second cardinal suture at 180° from the first is critical, ensuring equal distribution of tissue on either side of the diameter between the two sutures.

Suture Bites

Undue tension in sutures causes tissue compression and wound-related corneal steepening [2]. The longer and deeper the bites, the greater the volume of tissue that can be compressed, but the easier it is to control the tension. Sutures which are too loose or superficial favour wound gape and corneal flattening [5]. Some surgeons use continuous rather than interrupted sutures in the hope that the tension will be evenly distributed along the length of the wound [9, 35]. However, in practice, it is possible to create great variability in the tension of the suture and overtighten it or leave it too loose.

Suture Orientation
Sutures should be placed perpendicularly across an incision. For keratoplasty or cataract surgery, where the incision is parallel with the limbus, this means that the sutures should be radial. Sutures in any other orientation will tend to drag one wound edge relative to the other, resulting in horizontal misalignment.

Suture Material
Wounds sutured with silk or absorbable sutures (e.g. catgut, Vicryl) initially demonstrate wound-related steepening, which after 6–8 weeks converts to flattening as the sutures are degraded [1, 6, 36–40]. In contrast, monofilament nylon, which is an inert non-absorbable suture with a relatively high tensile strength, allows minimal natural decay of induced astigmatism, until the suture is removed [1, 3, 5, 8, 41–45]. Any natural decay which does occur is greatest in the first month postoperatively [21]. The use of well-constructed small (≤4 mm) self-sealing incisions avoids the use of sutures and their related complications [3] and is not associated with significant wound-related flattening [8, 25].

Intraoperative Topography
Keratoscopy can be performed intraoperatively using conical Placido rings viewed through a central hole, a circular plastic ring which focuses the microscope light on the cornea or a microscope-mounted ring of lights. Many surgeons advocate its use during the suturing of corneal wounds in order to reduce surgically induced astigmatism [46–49], but others are unconvinced of its value [50]. This latter view is supported by two explanations: firstly, the configuration of the globe during surgery may not be the same as postoperatively due to the speculum, abnormal intraocular pressure, etc. and, secondly, corneal topography changes spontaneously with healing during the months after surgery and when the sutures are removed. However, obtaining a symmetric corneal shape at the end of surgery is likely to provide more rapid visual rehabilitation.

Postoperative Factors

Corneal topography is useful following keratoplasty to identify tight sutures for removal, to determine the corneal component of a poor optical outcome and to plan astigmatic correction [12, 51–57] or cataract surgery [58] (Chap. 12), if required.

Suture Adjustment

In wounds closed by non-absorbable sutures, selective suture manipulation postoperatively is an effective way of reducing wound-related corneal steepening [59, 60]. For limbal and peripheral corneal incisions, this may be performed at 8–12 weeks postoperatively [61, 62], but for central corneal sutures [63] and following keratoplasty, it may not be safe to remove sutures for many months [61, 64]. In patients receiving topical corticosteroids, corneal wound healing is retarded, so suture removal should be delayed.

For interrupted sutures, those which are tight can be removed from the steep axis/axes at the appropriate time [61, 62], but the area of removal then tends to be flatter than the areas where sutures remain, and the axis of the astigmatism swings round. Unless there is one particularly tight suture, it is often more effective to remove all the sutures at the same time once the wound is sufficiently healed. Continuous sutures may be removed entirely [65], or alternatively the tension in the suture may be redistributed by easing it loop by loop from flat areas to steep areas [60, 66], but this risks breaking the suture. Corneal topography is of greater benefit than keratometry for suture adjustment following keratoplasty, because it will identify more accurately the location of the tight sutures, particularly if there is more than one.

References

*References Particularly Worth Reading

1. *Swinger CA. Postoperative astigmatism. Surv Ophthalmol. 1987;31:219–48.
2. *van Rij G, Waring GO III. Changes in corneal curvature induced by sutures and incisions. Am J Ophthalmol. 1984;98:773–83.
3. Minkovitz JB, Stark WJ. Corneal complications of intraocular surgery. Curr Opin Ophthalmol. 1995;6:79–85.
4. Koch DD, Haft EA, Gay C. Computerized videokeratographic analysis of corneal topographic changes induced by sutured and unsutured 4mm scleral pocket incisions. J Cataract Refract Surg. 1993;19(Suppl):166–9.
5. Eve FR, Troutman RC. Placement of sutures used in corneal incisions. Am J Ophthalmol. 1976;82:786–9.
6. Stainer GA, Binder PS, Parker WT, Perl T. The natural and modified course of postcataract astigmatism. Ophthalmic Surg. 1982;13:822–7.
7. Geggel HS. Effect of peripheral subepithelial fibrosis on corneal transplant topography. J Cataract Refract Surg. 1996;22:135–8.
8. Martin RG, Sanders DR, Miller JD, Cox CC, Ballew C. Effect of cataract wound incision size on acute changes in corneal topography. J Cataract Refract Surg. 1993;19(Suppl):170–7.
9. Iliff CE, Khodadoust A. Control of astigmatism in cataract surgery. Am J Ophthalmol. 1968;65:378–82.
10. *Tripoli NK, Ibrahim OS, Coggins JM, et al. Quantitative and qualitative topography classification of clear penetrating keratopathies. Invest Ophthalmol Vis Sci. 1990;30(Suppl):480.
11. *Karabatsas CH, Cook S, Sparrow JM. A proposed classification for topographic patterns seen after penetrating keratoplasty. Br J Ophthalmol. 1999;83(4):403–9.
12. Price NC, Steele AD. The correction of post-keratoplasty astigmatism. Eye. 1987;1:562–6.
13. Williams KA, Roder D, Esterman A, et al. Factors predictive of corneal graft survival: report from the Australian corneal graft registry. Ophthalmology. 1992;99(3):403–14.
14. Olson RJ, Pingree M, Ridges R, et al. Penetrating keratoplasty for keratoconus: a long-term review of results and complications. J Cataract Refract Surg. 2000;26(7):987–91.

15. Williams KA, Hornsby NB, Bartlett CM, et al. Report from the Australian corneal graft registry. Adelaide: Tech. Rep., Snap Printing; 2004.
16. Javadi MA, Motlagh BF, Jafarinasab MR, et al. Outcomes of penetrating keratoplasty in keratoconus. Cornea. 2005;24(8):941–6.
17. Troutman RC, Swinger CA. Relaxing incision for control of postoperative astigmatism following keratoplasty. Ophthalmic Surg. 1980;90:131–6.
18. Troutman RC, Gaster RN. Surgical advances and results of keratoconus. Am J Ophthalmol. 1980;90:131–6.
19. Chow SP, Hopkinson CL, Tole DT, et al. Stability of visual outcome between 2 and 5 years following corneal transplantation in the United Kingdom. Br J Ophthalmol. 2018;102(1):37–41.
20. Kwitko S, Garbus JJ, Hwang DG, Gauderman WJ, McDonnell PJ. Computer-assisted study of diurnal variation in corneal topography after penetrating keratoplasty. Ophthalmic Surg. 1992;23:10–6.
21. *Khong AM, Mannis MJ, Plotnik RD, Johnson CA. Computerised topographic analysis of the healing graft after penetrating keratoplasty for keratoconus. Am J Ophthalmol. 1993;115:209–15.
22. *Chern KC, Meiser DM, Wilson SE, Macsai MS, Krasney RH. Small-diameter, round, eccentric penetrating keratoplasties and corneal topographic correlation. Ophthalmology. 1997;104:643–7.
23. Girard LJ, Rodriguez J, Mailman ML. Reducing surgically induced astigmatism by using a scleral tunnel. Am J Ophthalmol. 1984;97:450–6.
24. Nielsen PJ. Prospective evaluation of surgically induced astigmatism and astigmatic keratotomy effects of various self-sealing small incisions. J Cataract Refract Surg. 1995;21:43–8.
25. Kohnen T. Corneal shape changes and astigmatic aspects of scleral and corneal tunnel incisions [editorial]. J Cataract Refract Surg. 1997;23:301–2.
26. Oshika T, Tsuboi S, Yaguchi S, Yoshitomi F, Nagamoto T, Nagahara K, Emi K. Comparative study of intraocular lens implantation through 3.2 and 5.5mm incisions. Ophthalmology. 1994;101:1183–90.
27. *Levy JH, Pisacano AM, Chadwick K. Astigmatic changes after cataract surgery with 5.1mm and 3.5mm sutureless incisions. J Cataract Refract Surg. 1994;20:630–3.
28. *Hayashi K, Hayashi H, Nakao F, Hayashi F. The correlation between incision size and corneal shape changes in sutureless cataract surgery. Ophthalmology. 1995;102:550–6.
29. Kohnen T, Dick B, Jacobi KW. Comparison of the induced astigmatism after temporal clear corneal tunnel incisions of different sizes. J Cataract Refract Surg. 1995;21:417–24.
30. Storr-Paulsen A, Henning V. Long-term astigmatic changes after phacoemulsification with single stitch, horizontal suture closure. J Cataract Refract Surg. 1995;21:429–32.
31. Long DA, Monica ML. A prospective evaluation of corneal curvature changes with 3.0- to 3.5-mm corneal tunnel phacoemulsification. Ophthalmology. 1996;103:226–32.
32. Vass C, Menapace R, Amon M, Hirsch U, Yousef A. Batch-by-batch analysis of topographic changes induced by sutured and sutureless clear corneal incisions. J Cataract Refract Surg. 1996;22:324–30.
33. Ernest PH. Corneal lip tunnel incision. J Cataract Refract Surg. 1994;20:154–7.
34. Vass C, Menapace R, Rainer G. Corneal topographic changes after frown and straight sclerocorneal incisions. J Cataract Refract Surg. 1997;23:913–22.
35. Filatov V, Alexandrakis G, Talamo JH, Steinert RF. Comparison of suture-in and suture-out postkeratoplasty astigmatism with single running suture or combined running and interrupted sutures. Am J Ophthalmol. 1996;122:696–700.
36. Gorn RA. Surgically induced corneal astigmatism and its spontaneous regression. Ophthalmic Surg. 1985;16:162–4.
37. Singh D, Kumar K. Keratometric changes after cataract extraction. Br J Ophthalmol. 1976;60:638–41.
38. Dowling JL. Wound closure in cataract surgery. Ophthalmic Surg. 1981;12:574–7.

39. Floyd G. Changes in the corneal curvature following cataract surgery. Am J Ophthalmol. 1951;34:1525–33.
40. Jaffe NS, Clayman HM. The pathophysiology of corneal astigmatism after cataract extraction. Trans Am Acad Ophthalmol Otolaryngol. 1975;79:615–30.
41. Wishart MS, Wishart PK, Gregor ZJ. Corneal astigmatism following cataract extraction. Br J Ophthalmol. 1986;70:825–30.
42. Kondrot EC. Keratometric cylinder and visual recovery following phacoemulsification and intraocular lens implantation using a self-sealing cataract incision. J Cataract Refract Surg. 1991;17(Suppl):731–3.
43. Talamo JH, Stark WJ, Gottsch JD, Goodman DF, Pratzer K, Cravy TV, Enger C. Natural history of corneal astigmatism after cataract surgery. J Cataract Refract Surg. 1991;17:313–8.
44. O'Driscoll AM, Goble RR, Hallack GN, Andrew NC. A prospective, controlled study of a 9/0 elastic polypropylene suture for cataract surgery: refractive results and complications. Eye. 1994;8:538–42.
45. Drews RC. Astigmatism after cataract surgery: nylon versus mersilene. J Cataract Refract Surg. 1995;21:70–2.
46. Serarevic ON, Renard GJ, Pouliquen Y. Randomised clinical trial comparing astigmatism and visual rehabilitation after penetrating keratoplasty with and without intraoperative suture adjustment. Ophthalmology. 1994;106:990–9.
47. Samples JR, Binder PS. The value of the Terry Keratometer in predicting postoperative astigmatism. Ophthalmology. 1984;91:280–4.
48. Morlet N. Clinical utility of the Barrett keratoscope with astigmatic dial. Ophthalmic Surg. 1994;25:150–3.
49. Thall EH, Lange SR. Preliminary results of a new intraoperative corneal topography technique. J Cataract Refract Surg. 1993;19(Suppl):193–7.
50. *Frantz JM, Reidy JJ, McDonald, MB. A comparison of surgical keratometers. Refract Corneal Surg. 1989;5:409–13.
51. *Maguire LJ, Bourne WM. Corneal topography of transverse keratotomies for astigmatism after penetrating keratoplasty. Am J Ophthalmol. 1989;107:323–30.
52. Krachmer JH, Fenzl RE. Surgical correction of high postkeratoplasty astigmatism: relaxing incisions vs wedge resection. Arch Ophthalmol. 1980;98:1400–2.
53. Sugar J, Kirk A. Relaxing keratotomy for post-keratoplasty high astigmatism. Ophthalmic Surg. 1983;14:156–8.
54. Lavery GW, Lindstrom RL, Hofer LA, Doughman DJ. The surgical management of corneal astigmatism after penetrating keratoplasty. Ophthalmic Surg. 1985;16:165–9.
55. Güell JL, Manero F, Müller A. Transverse keratotomy to correct high corneal astigmatism after cataract surgery. J Cataract Refract Surg. 1996;22:331–6.
56. Lazzaro DR, Haight DH, Belmont SC, Gibralter RP, Aslanides IM, Odrich MG. Excimer laser keratectomy for astigmatism occurring after penetrating keratoplasty. Ophthalmology. 1996;103:458–64.
57. Amm M, Duncker GIW, Schröder E. Excimer laser correction of high astigmatism after keratoplasty. J Cataract Refract Surg. 1996;22:313–7.
58. Serdarevic ON, Renard GJ, Pouliquen Y. Videokeratoscopy of recipient peripheral corneas in combined penetrating keratoplasty, cataract extraction, and lens implantation. Am J Ophthalmol. 1996;122:29–37.
59. *Strelow S, Cohen EJ, Leavitt KG, Laibson PR. Corneal topography for selective suture removal after penetrating keratoplasty. Am J Ophthalmol. 1991;112:657–65.
60. Roper-Hall MJ. Control of astigmatism after surgery and trauma. Br J Ophthalmol. 1982;66:556–9.
61. Kronish JW, Forster RK. Control of corneal astigmatism following cataract extraction by selective suture cutting. Arch Ophthalmol. 1987;105:1650–5.

62. Potamitis T, Fouladi M, Eperjese F, McDonnell PJ. Astigmatism decay immediately following suture removal. Eye. 1997;11:84–6.
63. *Navon SE. Topography after repair of full-thickness corneal laceration. J Cataract Refract Surg. 1997;23:495–501.
64. Binder PS. Selective suture removal can reduce postkeratoplasty astigmatism. Ophthalmology. 1985;92:1412–6.
65. Luntz MH, Livingstone DG. Astigmatism in cataract surgery. Br J Ophthalmol. 1977;61:360–5.
66. Atkins AD, Roper-Hall MJ. Control of postoperative astigmatism. Br J Ophthalmol. 1985;69:348–51.

Cataract Surgery

12

Cataract surgery is usually performed with the aim of improving vision. Over the years, technological advances have enabled a greater and greater degree of improvement to be achieved. Originally, surgeons concentrated on the removal of the opacified lens to enable light to enter the posterior portion of the globe. With the introduction of microsurgery and intraocular lenses, patients could hope for a return of good best-corrected visual acuity. Following the most recent developments in cataract surgery, attention has turned to ensuring that light is brought to an optimum focus on the retina, in order to provide patients with good uncorrected vision.

However, the lens contributes only one-third of the total focusing power of the eye. The remaining two-thirds arises from the convex shape of the anterior corneal surface. This has two important implications for cataract surgery. Firstly, knowledge of the power contributed by the cornea is essential to accurately calculate the power of intraocular lens to be inserted. Secondly, very small changes in corneal shape can have a dramatic effect on the precision with which light rays are brought to a focus on the retina. Therefore, incisions made in the cornea or anterior sclera during cataract extraction have the potential to change the refraction of the eye. Assessments of corneal topography can be used to minimise the adverse results of these incisions and even utilise their effects to advantage.

It has long been known that the surgical removal of cataracts can be associated with marked changes in corneal curvature, which can limit visual rehabilitation postoperatively [1, 2]. In 1864, before corneal sutures were available, Franz Donders reported the occurrence of "against-the-rule" astigmatism (flattening in the vertical meridian) following cataract extraction [3]. Keratometric measurements were subsequently documented by von Reuss and Woinow in 1869 [4]. For almost the next century, the basic techniques for cataract surgery changed little and were associated with significant ocular morbidity.

Over recent decades, there have been numerous changes, which have resulted in great improvements in efficacy. Intraocular lenses (IOLs) have been developed and refined, as have suture materials, surgical microscopes and micro-instrumentation. Techniques have evolved from intracapsular to extracapsular procedures and then to

© Springer Nature Switzerland AG 2019
M. Corbett et al., *Corneal Topography*,
https://doi.org/10.1007/978-3-030-10696-6_12

Table 12.1 Role of corneal topography in cataract surgery

Role of topography in cataract surgery	
Preoperative	Calculation of IOL power
	Planning the incision
	Location
	Length
	Architecture
Intraoperative	Suture adjustment (limited value)
Postoperative	Suture adjustment
	Investigation of a poor outcome
	Surgical correction of induced astigmatism

IOL intraocular lens

small-incision techniques with phacoemulsification and foldable lens implants. Cataract surgery is now routinely performed on a day case basis with rapid visual rehabilitation, little morbidity and high expectations of a successful outcome by both surgeons and patients alike.

Nowadays, the aim of cataract surgery is to return patients to good uncorrected vision. This requires that their final refraction should be within 0.5D of emmetropia or a predetermined ametropic result and that pre-existing and surgically induced astigmatism should be minimised [5, 6]. In order to achieve this, the refractive element of each stage of surgery has to be optimised. This is facilitated, particularly in difficult cases, by the use of corneal topography [7, 8] (Table 12.1).

Preoperative Topography

The preoperative assessment of corneal topography has two roles in cataract surgery (Fig. 12.1). Firstly, as an alternative to keratometry, it can provide a representative measure of corneal curvature or power, which is necessary for the calculation of IOL power. Secondly, knowledge of the magnitude and location of pre-existing astigmatism is important if it is to be reversed by (a) the appropriate placement and construction of the wound during surgery, (b) the insertion of a toric IOL or (c) postoperative "top-up" femtosecond or excimer laser correction.

Calculation of IOL Power

Prior to cataract surgery, the power of intraocular lens required to give the desired postoperative refraction is determined. This is most frequently done by using measurements of corneal power and axial length in a mathematical or theoretical formula [9–18]. There are several different formulas in use, but one of the original ones (and now obsolete) is the SRK formula:

$$P = A - 2.5L - 0.9K$$

Fig. 12.1 Role of topography in cataract surgery. In cases with irregular corneas, topography can improve the uncorrected visual outcome by increasing the accuracy of intraocular lens (IOL) power calculations and enabling the astigmatism to be addressed at the time of surgery

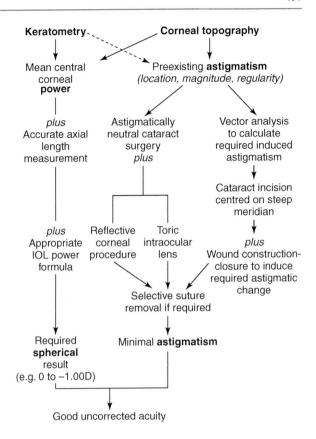

where *P* is the power of the intraocular lens required for emmetropia, *A* is a constant particular to each model of lens, *L* is the axial length of the eye (mm) and *K* is the keratometric power (*D*). The postoperative refraction in a given patient is dependent upon the accuracy of the biometric data and its appropriate use in the formula (Fig. 12.1). Newer-generation formulas (Barrett, Haigis, Hoffer Q, Holliday, SRK/T) take into account more parameters, such as anterior chamber depth (ACD), lens thickness, white-to-white corneal diameter, effective lens position and preoperative refraction to generate greater accuracy in predicting postoperative refraction [9–15]. Recently, the Hill-RBF calculator has been devised. It is a self-validating method of IOL power selection that utilises radial basis function and is entirely data-driven. Therefore, it is independent of the limitations of theoretical formulas which make assumptions regarding effective lens position [15].

The corneal curvature is commonly been measured by keratometry, with the mean of the two readings being used in the formula. For the majority of normal corneas, the small variability of the keratometry readings gives an accuracy of IOL power within the 0.5D step interval of manufactured lenses [19, 20]. In this group, variability in the measurement of the axial length tends to be the greatest source of discrepancy in the IOL power prediction [21]. For devices that measure both

Table 12.2 Alternative groups of topographic data points which could be used to generate the keratometric values in the formula to calculate the power of an intraocular lens

Data point options s
Keratometric equivalent at the 3 mm zone [813, 814] (average of the steepest and flattest meridians)
Average curvature of the 3 mm ring [800]
Average curvature of the 4 mm ring
Mean central corneal power 800]
Centrally weighted mean corneal power [461]

keratometry and axial length (such as the optically based biometers), it is usually preferable to use its own keratometry measurements if they are accurate, as the algorithms within the device are calibrated using those.

In contrast, this is not necessarily the case for patients who have corneal pathology or have undergone previous corneal or refractive procedures [7, 22–32]. When the cornea is irregular, a better prediction of the required IOL power can be obtained by using corneal topography than keratometry to measure the corneal curvature [19, 33]. As a result of generating many more data points, corneal topography has the advantage of representing these corneas more accurately; but with it comes the difficulty of knowing which data points to use in the IOL power calculations [19, 34] (Table 12.2). Moreover, different sets of data points may be most accurate with different formulas [15, 21]. On the whole, measurements using a greater number of data points from nearer the central cornea are most useful.

Planning the Incision

Knowledge of the magnitude, location and regularity of pre-existing astigmatism is important if it is to be reversed prior to or during cataract surgery (Fig. 12.1). Vector analysis can be used to calculate the induced astigmatism, which needs to be added to the existing astigmatism in order to produce the desired spherical end result [30, 35]. This may be achieved by three alternative methods [5, 36]. Firstly, astigmatic keratotomy may be performed prior to or during cataract surgery [37–39]. Secondly, a toric intraocular lens can be implanted. Thirdly, the astigmatism may be addressed by using the appropriate placement and construction of the incision [40]. This is done by centring the incision on the steep meridian and using a wound construction-closure combination that will produce the required astigmatic decay [41]. If sutures have been used, the effect can be further titrated against the topography by selective suture removal postoperatively.

Incision Location

Surgically induced changes in corneal contour are less following more peripheral (posterior) incisions in the sclera or limbus [22, 41, 42] than those involving the cornea. Some authors have claimed that for smaller incision surgery, some incision sites (e.g. superotemporal or temporal) cause less astigmatism than others [40, 43].

Incision Length

There is now a huge quantity of literature supporting the theory that smaller incisions are associated with less surgically induced change in corneal contour, a more stable refraction, earlier visual recovery and a better uncorrected visual acuity, particularly early after surgery [6, 44–51]. Since the introduction of intraocular lenses with flexible optics, it has been shown that an unsutured 2.0 mm incision is usually associated with less than 0.5D against-the-rule shift in corneal astigmatism.

Incision Architecture

Multiplanar incisions are commonly used to aid vertical alignment and give the wound greater stability. As incisions have become smaller, a tunnel construction has been introduced to make wounds self-sealing, thereby avoiding the need for sutures and the consequent suture-induced astigmatism [6, 40, 52, 53].

Wound Closure

Sutureless Incisions

The use of well-constructed self-sealing incisions avoids suture-related complications, and postoperative astigmatism is no longer the frequent and serious problem it used to be [6, 46, 48]. Unsutured small incision wounds typically show only a mild "against-the-rule" astigmatic shift (<1.00D) which tends to decay with time [15, 47, 51, 54] (Fig. 12.2). If flattening occurs, it tends to remain localised to the area of the wound, and does not necessarily reduce uncorrected visual acuity unless it encroaches on the central cornea (Fig. 12.3).

Sutured Wounds

If large (>5 mm) wounds require suturing, monofilament nylon is commonly used. This is an inert non-absorbable suture with a relatively high tensile strength, which allows minimal natural decay of induced astigmatism (Figs. 12.4 and 12.5), until the suture is removed [55–59]. For small incisions (<5 mm), a thin monofilament absorbable suture such as Vicryl is often used as it will disintegrate in about 1 month.

To minimise surgically induced astigmatism, radial sutures should be relatively deep and of moderate length to prevent tissue compression or wound gape [2, 55] (Chap. 11). For tunnel incisions, some studies suggest that horizontal, triangular or mattress sutures are associated with less wound-related steepening than either radial or cross sutures [5, 22, 60].

Topography After Cataract Surgery

The topographic changes induced as a result of cataract surgery are similar to those induced by other surgery in the peripheral cornea or at the limbus such as endothelial transplantation and can therefore be used as a model for describing those changes. Any changes induced during surgery can be displayed using a "change" or "difference" map which compares two maps, by subtracting the preoperative measurements from the postoperative measurements [34] (Chap. 5). As most of the primary changes relate to the incision site in the corneal periphery, they are shown to

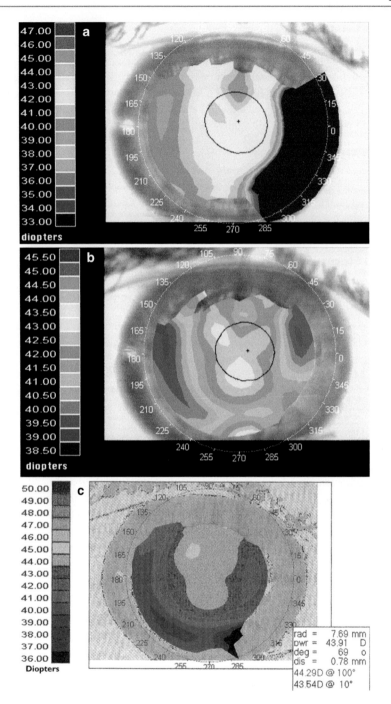

Fig. 12.2 Small incision flattening. A patient with oval-pattern topography underwent phaco-emulsification through an unsutured superior 3.2 mm clear corneal tunnel of length 2 mm. (**a**) One week postoperatively, there was localised flattening associated with the incision and just extending into the pupillary aperture. However, the central cornea remained regular, and there was less than half a dioptre of astigmatism. (**b**) By 3 months, the flattening was reducing and was largely outside the pupillary zone. (**c**) At 1 year, the topography was regular again. Note the difference in the scales

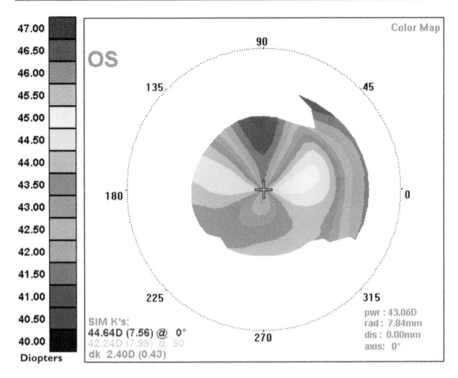

Fig. 12.3 Large incision flattening. Following extracapsular cataract extraction through a 12 mm incision which is sutured too loosely, the induced corneal flattening involves the central cornea. In this case, 2.40DC astigmatism has been generated

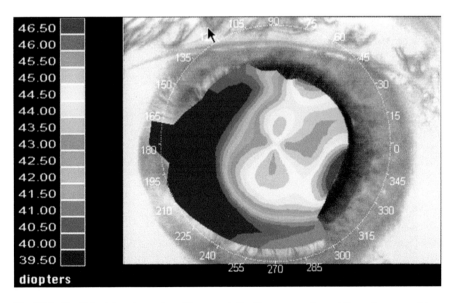

Fig. 12.4 Small incision steepening. Phacoemulsification was performed through a corneal tunnel. This was closed by a single X-suture at 65° which induced 2D of corneal astigmatism. There was local peripheral steepening associated with the paracentesis at 340°, which settled rapidly

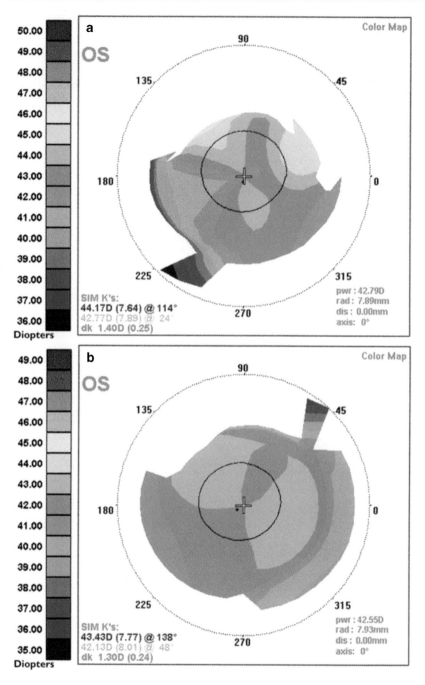

Fig. 12.5 Large incision steepening. Following extracapsular cataract extraction, the 12 mm incision was closed with five interrupted nylon sutures. (**a**) The sutures at 40° and 130° were too tight, producing focal steepening in these semimeridian and irregular (bi-oblique) astigmatisms. Refraction or keratometry alone identified the steep axis at 115° and the flat axis at 25°. This would have identified the wrong suture for removal in the nasal cornea and overlooked the tight suture in the temporal cornea. (**b**) Once the tight sutures were removed, the cornea reverted to a regular pattern which could be corrected by a spherocylindrical lens

Table 12.3 Classification of the topographic changes induced by cataract surgery [465, 763]

Topographic changes induced by cataract surgery	
Location	Magnitude
Central	>1D, within the central 2×2 mm
Peripheral	>1D, away from the wound
Wound-related	Extending to within:
1+	Central 7 mm
2+	Central 5 mm
3+	Central 3 mm
Astigmatic	Increase or decrease by >1DC

best advantage if the scale used is local rather than global radius of curvature. These primary changes may induce secondary changes in the perpendicular meridian as a result of "coupling" (Chap. 9).

Surgery can result in either steepening or flattening of one or more parts of the cornea (Chap. 11). These changes can be classified according to their location relative to the wound and their magnitude [44, 46] (Table 12.3).

Corneal Steepening

Wound-related corneal steepening (with-the-rule astigmatism for a superior incision) occurs secondary to compression of tissue at the wound site [1] (Figs. 12.4 and 12.5). This is commonly a result of the overtightening of sutures or oedema of the wound margin. It may also be due to vertical wound malalignment in which the central edge under-rides the peripheral edge or due to cautery causing tissue contraction [22] (Fig. 11.1).

The compression of tissue at the limbus depresses the peripheral cornea towards the centre of the globe, thereby increasing the curvature of the central cornea (i.e. a reduction in the radius of curvature) [2]. There is a small area of flattening immediately within the area of the suture and a secondary flattening in the meridian perpendicular to the suture, as a result of coupling.

Corneal Flattening

Wound-related corneal flattening (against-the-rule astigmatism for a superior incision) occurs as a result of wound gape [1, 2] (Figs. 12.2 and 12.3). This is sometimes seen to a small extent in unsutured wounds [22, 47, 51, 54] but more commonly if sutures are too loose either at the time of surgery or if there is subsequent cheese-wiring, knot-slippage, suture-related inflammation, degradation or removal. Sutures which are placed too superficially may result in posterior wound gape, which has a similar topographic appearance. Vertical misalignment of the wound with the central edge over-riding the peripheral edge also produces wound-related corneal flattening (Fig. 11.1). If the wound edges are in poor apposition and the gaping area is filled by fibrovascular scar tissue, this may later stretch leading to increased corneal flattening.

Wound gape increases the circumference of the globe in the meridian perpendicular to the line of the incision, thereby flattening the incisional meridian [2].

Irregular Astigmatism

If wound-related flattening or steepening is due to either a single or a uniform structural defect, regular astigmatism is most likely and is relatively easy to correct either optically or surgically. However, more complex anatomical changes can result in irregular astigmatism, which produces greater visual dysfunction and is more difficult to correct [60]. Bi-oblique astigmatism (non-perpendicular axes) may occur if nonadjacent sutures are overtightened (Figs. 11.1 and 12.5). A torsional effect results from a horizontal misalignment of the wound, whether due to a mismatching of its edges or non-radial suture bites (Figs. 11.1 and 12.6).

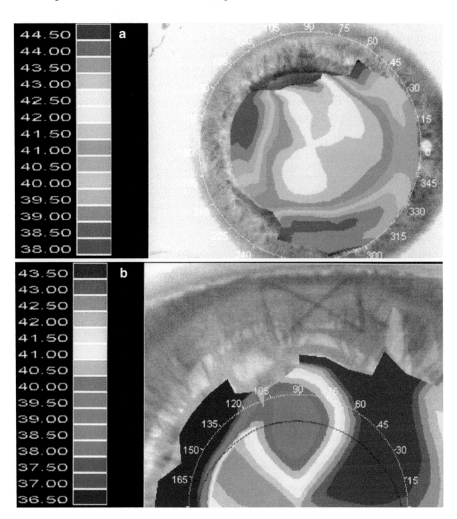

Fig. 12.6 Wound misalignment. Following left phacoemulsification through a 5.5 mm incision, horizontal mismatching of the wound edges has given the topography a torsional appearance, resulting in irregular astigmatism (**a**). The zoomed view (**b**) shows that the single X-suture has dragged the central edge of the wound nasally with respect to the limbus. A similar effect occurs if the suture bites are not radial

Postoperative Topography

Postoperatively, corneal topography or keratometry can be used routinely to identify tight sutures that should be removed. Topography is valuable in patients with an inadequate best-corrected visual acuity, in order to determine whether corneal irregularities account for the poor level of vision. In patients who require surgical correction of a persisting refractive error or irregular astigmatism, corneal topography is essential.

Suture Adjustment

In wounds closed by non-absorbable sutures, selective suture manipulation at 12 weeks postoperatively is an effective way of reducing wound-related corneal steepening. For interrupted sutures, this involves removal of the tight suture(s) in the steep axis/axes [61, 62]. For continuous, the tension in the suture may be redistributed by easing it loop by loop from flat areas to steep areas [63, 64], but this risks breaking the suture so is seldom performed these days.

Corneal topography is of greater benefit than keratometry for suture adjustment, because it will identify more accurately the location of the tight sutures, particularly if more than one is tight (Fig. 12.5).

Investigation of Poor Outcome

Corneal topography should be performed after cataract surgery in cases in which the best-corrected visual acuity is not adequate, and there are no other obvious causes for poor vision [64]. It will determine whether there are irregularities of the corneal surface and whether they are amenable to correction [6, 33].

Surgical Correction of Postoperative Astigmatism

Postoperative astigmatism persisting after suture removal can be addressed either by revision of the original incision or a separate corneal refractive procedure [5] (Chap. 13).

References

* References Particularly Worth Reading

1. *Swinger CA. Postoperative astigmatism. Surv Ophthalmol. 1987;31:219–48.
2. *van Rij G, Waring GO III. Changes in corneal curvature induced by sutures and incisions. Am J Ophthalmol. 1984;98:773–83.

 3. Donders F. On the anomalies of refraction and accommodation of the eye. London: The New Sydenham Society; 1864.
 4. von ReussWoinow. Ophthalmometrische Studien. Wein; 1869.
 5. *Nordan LT, Lusby FW. Refractive aspects of cataract surgery. Curr Opin Ophthalmol. 1995;6:36–40.
 6. *Minkovitz JB, Stark WJ. Corneal complications of intraocular surgery. Curr Opin Ophthalmol. 1995;6:79–85.
 7. *Martinez CE, Klyce SD. Corneal topography in cataract surgery. Curr Opin Ophthalmol. 1996;7:31–8.
 8. Thornton SP. Clinical evaluation of corneal topography. J Cataract Refract Surg. 1993;19(Suppl):198–202.
 9. Sanders DR, Retzlaff J, Kraff MC. Comparison of the SRK II″ formula and other second generation formulas. J Cataract Refract Surg. 1988;14:136–41.
10. Holladay JT. Standardizing constants for ultrasonic biometry, keratometry, and intraocular lens power calculations. J Cataract Refract Surg. 1997;23(9):1356–70.
11. Haigis VV. The Haigis formula. Chap 5. In: Shammas H, editor. Intraocular lens power calculations. Thorofare: Slack; 2003. p. 41–57.
12. Hoffer KJ. The Hoffer Q formula: a comparison of theoretic and regression formulas. J Cataract Refract Surg. 1993;19:700–12.
13. Melles RB, Holladay JT, Chang WJ. Accuracy of intraocular lens calculation formulas. Ophthalmology. 2018;125(2):169–78.
14. Koch DD, Hill W, Albulafia A, et al. Pursuing perfection in intraocular lens calculations: I. Logical approach for classifying IOL calculation formulas. JCRS. 2017;43(6):717–8.
15. Barrett GD. Barrett universal II formula. Singapore: Asia-Pacific Association of Cataract and Refractive Surgeons. Available at: http://www.apacrs.org/barrett_universal2/. Accessed 5 Jul 2016.
16. Ascaso FJ, Castillo JM, Cristobal JA, Minguez E, Palomar A. A comparative study of eight intraocular lens calculation formulas. Ophthalmologica. 1991;203:148–53.
17. Barrett GD. An improved universal theoretical formula for intraocular lens power prediction. J Cataract Refract Surg. 1993;19:713–20.
18. Hoffer KJ. The Hoffer Q formula: comparison of theoretic and regression formulas. J Cataract Refract Surg. 1993;19:700–12.
19. *Cuaycong MJ, Gay CA, Emery J, Haft EA, Koch DD. Comparison of the accuracy of computerized videokeratoscopy and keratometry for use in intraocular lens calculations. J Cataract Refract Surg. 1993;19(Suppl):178–81.
20. Husain SE, Kohnen T, Maturi R, Er H, Koch DD. Computerised videokeratography and keratometry in determining intraocular lens calculations. J Cataract Refract Surg. 1996;22:362–6.
21. Hovding G, Natvik C, Sletteberg O. The refractive error after implantation of a posterior chamber intraocular lens. The accuracy of IOL power calculation in a hospital practice. Acta Ophthalmol. 1994;72:612–6.
22. *Koch DD, Haft EA, Gay C. Computerized videokeratographic analysis of corneal topographic changes induced by sutured and unsutured 4mm scleral pocket incisions. J Cataract Refract Surg. 1993;19(Suppl):166–9.
23. McDonnell PJ. Can we avoid an epidemic of refractive 'surprises' after cataract surgery? [editorial]. Arch Ophthalmol. 1997;115:542–3.
24. Celikkol L, Ahn D, Celikkol G, Feldman ST. Calculating intraocular lens power in eyes with keratoconus using videokeratography. J Cataract Refract Surg. 1996;22:497–500.
25. Serdarevic ON, Renard GJ, Pouliquen Y. Videokeratoscopy of recipient peripheral corneas in combined penetrating keratoplasty, cataract extraction, and lens implantation. Am J Ophthalmol. 1996;122:29–37.
26. Flowers CW, MdLeod SD, McDonnell PJ, Irvine JA, Smith RE. Evaluation of intraocular lens power calculation formulas in the triple procedure. J Cataract Refract Surg. 1996;22:116–22.
27. Koch DD, Liu JF, Hyde LL, Rock RL, Emery JM. Refractive complications of cataract surgery after radial keratotomy. Am J Ophthalmol. 1989;108:676–82.

28. *Hoffer KJ. Intraocular lens power calculation for eyes after refractive keratotomy. J Refract Surg. 1995;11:490–3.
29. Lyle WA, Jin GJC. Intraocular lens power prediction in patients who undergo cataract surgery following previous radial keratotomy. Arch Ophthalmol. 1997;115:457–61.
30. Lesher MP, Schumer DJ, Hunkeler JD, Durrie DS, McKee FE. Phacoemulsification with intraocular lens implantation after excimer photorefractive keratectomy: a case report. J Cataract Refract Surg. 1994;20(Suppl):265–7.
31. Siganos DS, Pallikaris IG, Lambropoulos JE, Koufala CJ. Keratometric readings after photorefractive keratectomy are unreliable for calculating IOL power. J Refract Surg. 1996;12:S278–9.
32. Kalski RS, Danjoux J-P, Fraenkel GE, Lawless MA, Rogers C. Intraocular lens power calculation for cataract surgery after photorefractive keratectomy for high myopia. J Refract Surg. 1997;13:362–6.
33. Sanders RD, Gills JP, Martin RG. When keratometric measurements do not accurately reflect corneal topography. J Cataract Refract Surg. 1993;19(Suppl):131–5.
34. Vass C, Menapace R. Computerised statistical analysis of corneal topography for the evaluation of changes in corneal shape after surgery. Am J Ophthalmol. 1994;118:177–84.
35. Holladay JT, Cravy TV, Koch DD. Calculation of surgically induced refractive change following ocular surgery. J Cataract Refract Surg. 1992;18:429–43.
36. *Kohnen T, Koch DD. Control of astigmatism in cataract surgery. Curr Opin Ophthalmol. 1996;7:75–80.
37. Hall GW, Campion M, Sorenson CM, Monthofer S. Reduction of corneal astigmatism at cataract surgery. J Cataract Refract Surg. 1991;17:407–14.
38. Kershner RM. Keratolenticuloplasty: arcuate keratotomy for cataract surgery and astigmatism. J Cataract Refract Surg. 1995;21(and comments in J Cat Refract Surg 1995; 21: 597-8):274–7.
39. Masket S. Arcuate keratotomy for cataract surgery and astigmatism [letter]. J Cataract Refract Surg. 1995;21:597–8.
40. *Nielsen PJ. Prospective evaluation of surgically induced astigmatism and astigmatic keratotomy effects of various self-sealing small incisions. J Cataract Refract Surg. 1995;21:43–8.
41. Kohnen T. Corneal shape changes and astigmatic aspects of scleral and corneal tunnel incisions [editorial]. J Cataract Refract Surg. 1997;23:301–2.
42. Girard LJ, Rodriguez J, Mailman ML. Reducing surgically induced astigmatism by using a scleral tunnel. Am J Ophthalmol. 1984;97:450–6.
43. Hayashi K, Nakao F, Hayashi F. Corneal topographic analysis of superolateral incision cataract surgery. J Cataract Refract Surg. 1994;20:392–9.
44. *Martin RG, Sanders DR, Miller JD, Cox CC, Ballew C. Effect of cataract wound incision size on acute changes in corneal topography. J Cataract Refract Surg. 1993;19(Suppl):170–7.
45. Levy JH, Pisacano AM, Chadwick K. Astigmatic changes after cataract surgery with 5.1mm and 3.5mm sutureless incisions. J Cataract Refract Surg. 1994;20:630–3.
46. Oshika T, Tsuboi S, Yaguchi S, Yoshitomi F, Nagamoto T, Nagahara K, Emi K. Comparative study of intraocular lens implantation through 3.2 and 5.5mm incisions. Ophthalmology. 1994;101:1183–90.
47. Feil SH, Crandall AS, Olson RJ. Astigmatic decay following small incision, self-sealing cataract surgery. J Cataract Refract Surg. 1994;20:40–3.
48. *Hayashi K, Hayashi H, Nakao F, Hayashi F. The correlation between incision size and corneal shape changes in sutureless cataract surgery. Ophthalmology. 1995;102:550–6.
49. Kohnen T, Dick B, Jacobi KW. Comparison of the induced astigmatism after temporal clear corneal tunnel incisions of different sizes. J Cataract Refract Surg. 1995;21:417–24.
50. Long DA, Monica ML. A prospective evaluation of corneal curvature changes with 3.0- to 3.5-mm corneal tunnel phacoemulsification. Ophthalmology. 1996;103:226–32.
51. Pfleger T, Skorpik C, Menapace R, Scholz U, Weghaupt H, Zehetmayer M. Long-term course of induced astigmatism after clear corneal incision cataract surgery. J Cataract Refract Surg. 1996;22:72–7.
52. Ernest PH. Corneal lip tunnel incision. J Cataract Refract Surg. 1994;20:154–7.

53. Vass C, Menapace R, Rainer G. Corneal topographic changes after frown and straight sclero-corneal incisions. J Cataract Refract Surg. 1997;23:913–22.
54. Vass C, Menapace R, Amon M, Hirsch U, Yousef A. Batch-by-batch analysis of topographic changes induced by sutured and sutureless clear corneal incisions. J Cataract Refract Surg. 1996;22:324–30.
55. Eve FR, Troutman RC. Placement of sutures used in corneal incisions. Am J Ophthalmol. 1976;82:786–9.
56. Wishart MS, Wishart PK, Gregor ZJ. Corneal astigmatism following cataract extraction. Br J Ophthalmol. 1986;70:825–30.
57. O'Driscoll AM, Goble RR, Hallack GN, Andrew NC. A prospective, controlled study of a 9/0 elastic polypropylene suture for cataract surgery: refractive results and complications. Eye. 1994;8:538–42.
58. Drews RC. Astigmatism after cataract surgery: nylon versus mersilene. J Cataract Refract Surg. 1995;21:70–2.
59. Potamitis T, Fouladi M, Eperjese F, McDonnell PJ. Astigmatism decay immediately following suture removal. Eye. 1997;11:84–6.
60. Olsen T, Dam-Johansen M, Beke T, Hjortdal JO. Evaluating surgically induced astigmatism by Fourier analysis of corneal topography data. J Cataract Refract Surg. 1996;22:318–23.
61. Luntz MH, Livingstone DG. Astigmatism in cataract surgery. Br J Ophthalmol. 1977;61:360–5.
62. Kronish JW, Forster RK. Control of corneal astigmatism following cataract extraction by selective suture cutting. Arch Ophthalmol. 1987;105:1650–5.
63. Roper-Hall MJ. Control of astigmatism after surgery and trauma. Br J Ophthalmol. 1982;66:556–9.
64. Atkins AD, Roper-Hall MJ. Control of postoperative astigmatism. Br J Ophthalmol. 1985;69:348–51.
63. Lakshminarayanan V, Enoch JM, Raasch T, Crawford B, Nydaard RW. Refractive changes induced by intraocular lens tilt and longitudinal displacement. Arch Ophthalmol. 1986;104:90–2.
64. Güell JL, Manero F, Müller A. Transverse keratotomy to correct high corneal astigmatism after cataract surgery. J Cataract Refract Surg. 1996;22:331–6.

Refractive Corneal Surgery

13

For many centuries, the only widely available means of correcting refractive errors has been by spectacles. However, for over 100 years, ophthalmologists have been searching for a surgical method to permanently alter the refractive power of the eye [1]. Most work has concentrated on altering the shape of the cornea, as this is easily accessible, and contributes two-thirds of the total refractive power of the eye. The ability to successfully alter the refractive power of the cornea depends partly upon a detailed knowledge of its topography.

The alternative to refractive surgery performed on the cornea is intraocular lens implantation (Chap. 12). However, whether this procedure is performed alone or in combination with either clear lens extraction or cataract extraction, it has the risks associated with any intraocular procedure. The advantage of lenticular procedures is that relatively large alterations in refractive power can be achieved [2]. In contrast, corneal procedures are most accurate and predictable when used to correct small refractive errors. Therefore, high degrees of ametropia may be best corrected primarily using a lenticular procedure, and then minor refractive adjustments can be made subsequently to the cornea if necessary [3].

Mechanisms

A myopic eye is one which is unduly long for its refractive power. The majority of surgical techniques for correcting myopia aim to reduce the refractive power of the cornea by flattening its anterior surface (increasing the radius of curvature). In hyperopia, the reverse is true, and corrective refractive procedures aim to steepen (decrease the radius of curvature) of the anterior corneal surface. Astigmatism is corrected by altering the refractive effect in the appropriate meridian.

Corneal refractive surgery is effective through one of two mechanisms: firstly by altering the shape of the whole thickness of the corneal stroma or secondly by affecting only the anterior corneal surface.

M. Corbett et al., *Corneal Topography*,
https://doi.org/10.1007/978-3-030-10696-6_13

The stress equilibria in the collagen lamellae can be altered by either incisions traversing the full thickness of the corneal stroma (e.g. radial keratotomy, astigmatic keratotomy) or by applying persistent mechanical forces (e.g. intrastromal corneal rings). This results in a change in the configuration of the cornea which affects both its anterior and posterior surfaces (*this chapter*).

In contrast, in surface procedures, tissue is either added to the anterior corneal surface (e.g. epikeratophakia [4]), removed (e.g. keratectomy and excimer or femtosecond laser procedures) [5] or structurally altered (laser thermokeratoplasty) [6]. In these procedures, the integrity of the deep corneal stroma is maintained, and the shape of the posterior corneal surface remains unaltered (Chap. 14).

Role of Topography

As in other forms of corneal surgery (Chaps. 11 and 12), topography is valuable in the preoperative assessment and planning and postoperative monitoring and management of refractive procedures [7] (Table 13.1). However, there are three additional roles which are particularly useful in these cases.

Topographic maps can be helpful in the education of patients about the shape of their cornea, how it differs from normality, the changes occurring postoperatively and the source of optical problems they may have.

Topography can also educate surgeons, both in general terms and by demonstrating the effects of individual procedures they have performed. They aid communication between colleagues by providing a visual description of the shape of a cornea.

In an age of increasing medical litigation, corneal maps provide objective documentary evidence of the changes in corneal shape which have occurred. Ideally, all

Table 13.1 Role of corneal topography in refractive surgery

Role of topography in refractive surgery	
Preoperative	Screening for ocular disease
	Keratoconus
	Contact lens-induced corneal warpage
	Planning the surgery
	Incision location, length, depth
Intraoperative	Real-time monitoring
	Currently of limited value, ? useful in future
Postoperative	Documentation of immediate effects of surgery
	Assessment of healing
	Investigation of a poor outcome
	Planning of augmentation
	Biometry for cataract surgery
Throughout	Patient education
	Communication with colleagues
	Documentation for medicolegal purposes

patients undergoing refractive procedures should have preoperative topography and their first postoperative map taken as early as 1 week after surgery. This enables the changes induced by the surgeon to be distinguished from those occurring subsequently as a result of wound healing, injury or further intervention.

Preoperative Assessment for Refractive Surgery

Corneal topography is only one of the many steps which are essential in the preoperative assessment of patients undergoing refractive surgery (Table 13.2). In this group, particular importance must be attached to the social and psychological

Table 13.2 Preoperative evaluation of patients undergoing refractive surgery

Preoperative evaluation for refractive surgery		
History	Refractive	Spectacle wear
		Contact lens wear
		Prescriptions from the last few years
		Problems
	Ocular	Amblyopia
		Ocular disease
		Ocular surgery
	Medical	Past medical history
		Current medical problems
		Treatment history
	Social	Occupation
		Hobbies, sport, leisure
		Smoking, substance abuse
	Psychological	Personality
		Expectations
Examination	Vision	Unaided vision
		Best-corrected acuity
		Pinhole acuity
		Contrast sensitivity[a]
		Night vision[a], halos[a]
	Refraction	
	Biometry	Corneal topography
		Axial length[a]
	Slit lamp	Anterior segment biomicroscopy
		Tonometry
		Pupil size in dim illumination
	Pachymetry[b]	
	Specular microscopy[a]	
	Fundoscopy	Disc
		Macula
		Peripheral retina

[a]Preferable, but not essential
[b]Not required for surface laser ablation

aspects of the history to assess the suitability of patients for surgery. During the examination, fundoscopy to exclude vitreoretinal lesions is just as important as the assessment of the vision, refraction and anterior segment. Adequate counselling and informed consent is also essential prior to surgery.

Preoperative Screening

Preoperative corneal topography is useful for detecting two of the contraindications for refractive surgery, namely, refractive instability and pre-existing corneal disease. Stability of refraction is required prior to surgery to ensure that the appropriate correction is performed. Corneal disease should be excluded to reduce the likelihood of an unusual wound healing response or postoperative progression of a refractive problem (Fig. 14.8) [5, 8].

In patients presenting for the surgical correction of myopia, as many as 33% have abnormal corneal topography [10]. This has been found to be due to keratoconus in 6% of patients [10, 11] and corneal warpage in 38% of contact lens wearers [10]. In the majority of cases, the abnormality was not evident on inspection of the cornea or the Placido image but could be detected by corneal topography, stressing the importance of performing this investigation preoperatively.

Many patients with severe topographic abnormalities would be automatically excluded from refractive surgery, but for others with only very mild changes, such as subclinical keratoconus (Chap. 10), the surgeon will need detailed topographic information to aid the decision as to whether to proceed. Some studies have suggested that in subclinical keratoconus, both RK±AK [12] and PRK [13, 14] give similar results to those seen in normal patients, at least in the short term.

Many topographic patterns can result from contact lens-induced corneal warpage, but they tend to comprise flattening in the areas of lens-bearing, with possible adjacent steepening (Table 7.2). The changes are most severe and persistent in wearers of hard or rigid gas permeable lenses. After cessation of lens wear, the cornea tends to return to its former shape, with the greatest changes occurring early. A normal corneal shape usually returns within about a month following soft lens wear, although there is great individual variation. However, for rigid lenses, normality may not be reached for 5 months or more, and in some patients, stabilisation occurs with an abnormal pattern persisting [15, 16].

It has been suggested the minimum delay between the removal of contact lenses and the preoperative assessment should be 2 weeks for soft lenses and 4 weeks for hard and rigid gas permeable lenses [17]. If abnormalities persist after the cessation of lens wear, topography should be repeated at intervals until the corneal shape has normalised or stabilised.

It is possible to distinguish between contact lens-induced warpage and true keratoconus: they exhibit similar topography patterns (superior flattening and inferior steepening) but demonstrate different geometric shapes that can be readily differentiated [18].

The overall efficacy and safety of refractive surgery can be improved by preoperative topographic screening to exclude unpredictable variables such as contact lens-induced corneal warpage and occult ectatic disease [8, 9].

Preoperative Planning

Corneal topography is essential before all refractive procedures, to enable the surgeon to understand the refractive status of an individual eye and plan the optimum treatment for it. In addition, if a patient is unable to co-operate sufficiently to enable topography to be undertaken, for example, if they are too photophobic, then it should be considered whether they should be undergoing routine refractive surgery.

Indices

Several indices have been developed to help the clinician distinguish normal corneas from those with early or established pathology. These are based on pachymetry, anterior corneal curvature and elevation data.

Randleman Ectasia Risk Score System

A risk factor stratification scale has been devised to help clinicians more accurately predict the risk of ectasia following refractive laser procedures [19] (Tables 13.3 and 13.4). In a group of patients with postsurgical ectasia, assessment was made of preoperative, perioperative and postoperative characteristics (age, gender spherical equivalent refraction, pachymetry, topographic patterns, type of surgery performed, flap thickness, ablation depth, residual stromal bed thickness and postoperative date of ectasia diagnosis).

Table 13.3 The different parameters and scoring points of the Randleman Ectasia Risk Factor Scoring system [19]

Randleman ectasia risk factor score system					
	Points				
Parameter points	4	3	2	1	0
Topography pattern	FFC	Inferior steepening/ SRA		ABT	Normal/ SBT
RSB thickness (microns)	<240	240–259	260–279	280–299	>300
Age (years)		18–21	22–25	26–29	>30
CCT (microns)	<450	451–480	481–510		>510
MRSE	>−14	>−12 to −14	>−10 to −12	>−8 to −10	−8 or less

ABT asymmetric bow tie, *CCT* preoperative central corneal thickness, *D* dioptres, *FFKC* forme fruste keratoconus, *MRSE* preoperative manifest refraction spherical equivalent, *RSB* residual stromal bed, *SBT* symmetric bow tie, *SRA* skewed radial axis

Table 13.4 The cumulative risk scores and recommendations from the Randleman Ectasia Risk Factor Scoring system [19]

Randleman ectasia risk factor score categories		
Cumulative risk score	Risk category	Recommendations
0–2	Low	Proceed with LASIK or surface ablation
3	Moderate	Proceed with caution
4 or more	High	Do not perform laser refractive surgery

Percentage Tissue Altered (PTA) Index

This index assesses the association between the percentage of tissue altered and the risk of ectasia [20]. It is calculated using the following equation:

$$PTA = \frac{(FT + AF)}{CCT}$$

PTA = percent of tissue altered
FT = flap thickness
AD = ablation depth
CCT = preoperative central corneal thickness

This formula is a precise method for assessing ectasia risk, and PTA values below 40.0% correlate with the low incidence of ectasia.

Intraoperative Assessment

Intraoperative topography is seldom performed during refractive surgery, because the shape achieved at the end of surgery usually undergoes further changes postoperatively.

Postoperative Assessment

The postoperative regional variations in curvature across the corneal surface are best displayed by maps using local (instantaneous/tangential) radius of curvature (Fig. 1.2). These avoid the spherical bias inherent in maps using global (axial/sagittal) radius of curvature (Fig. 5.6).

Changes in corneal topography are shown to best effect by the use of difference maps, in which a latter map is subtracted from an earlier one [10, 50] (Fig. 5.15). The result of the surgery itself is demonstrated by subtraction of the immediate postoperative map from the preoperative one. The stability of the change, and the effect of the ensuing wound healing process, is quantified by the difference between a map taken soon after surgery and one taken subsequently.

The regularity and symmetry of the corneal surface can be observed on the map and can be quantified by the calculation of statistical indices (e.g. surface regularity index, SRI; surface asymmetry index, SAI) [21, 22] (Table 5.7). These indices, and most particularly the SRI, correlate well with visual performance.

In cases with a poor visual outcome, topography may detect surface anomalies which are not readily appreciated on biomicroscopic examination [23]. These include surface irregularities and small or decentred treatment zones [24–26]. If patients require contact lenses, topography is helpful for their fitting [27].

Planning of Further Surgery

Preoperative corneal topography is even more important for refractive enhancements than it is for primary procedures. It is also valuable in patients presenting for cataract extraction after refractive surgery, when keratometry is not sufficiently accurate for calculating the power of intraocular lens required [28–35] (Chap. 12).

Topography After Refractive Surgery

Refractive corneal procedures are performed with the aim of altering the curvature of the central cornea and usually have minimal effect on the corneal periphery. The area bearing the full intended correction is the optical zone. This tends to be surrounded by an intermediate zone of altered curvature, before normal cornea is reached in the periphery.

The natural corneal shape is aspheric and radially asymmetric: the radius of curvature changes from centre to limbus and does so at different rates along different semimeridians. The profile of the normal cornea along any meridian is prolate, meaning that it is steeper in the centre and becomes flattened towards the periphery (positive shape factor) (Table 6.2).

Refractive surgery changes the curvature of the central optical zone more than the periphery, so the asphericity of the cornea is altered. Treatments for hyperopia steepen the optical zone, so the cornea becomes increasingly prolate. Myopic treatments flatten the optical zone making the cornea less prolate or even oblate (flatter in the centre than in the periphery). This is most marked following radial keratotomy, in which the central flattening is associated with increased steepening in the midperiphery.

Effects of Topography on Visual Function

Optimal visual performance after refractive surgery is achieved by producing a uniform change in corneal curvature over a relatively large area, centred on the pupil [36–42].

Minor degrees of optical zone decentration and corneal surface irregularity may not necessarily reduce Snellen visual acuity [43–47] but can adversely affect more subtle aspects of visual function, detectable on contrast sensitivity testing [24, 48, 49] or ray-tracing analysis [42, 43], and induce astigmatism [26, 44, 45].

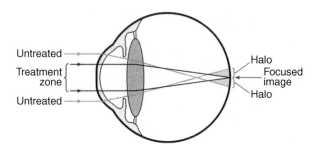

Fig. 13.1 Mechanism of halo formation. After refractive surgery with small optical zones, halos arise as a result of pupillary dilation in dim illumination. Under such conditions, the retinal image formed by focused light passing through the optical zone is degraded by unfocused light passing through the untreated peripheral cornea

More severe topographic anomalies can further degrade the retinal image leading to a reduction in Snellen acuity [46–48] and produce unwanted optical aberrations [49] including distortion, ghost images, halos (Fig. 13.1) and monocular diplopia [24, 50–53].

However, it has been suggested that the regional variations in corneal power resulting from radial keratotomy may explain why some patients achieve a visual acuity that is better than would be expected on the basis of their refractive error [54].

Radial Keratotomy

Radial keratotomy as such is seldom performed nowadays as it has been superseded by various forms of refractive laser surgery. However the principles of their topographic changes are applicable to other types of corneal incisions and trauma and can therefore guide decision-making in those situations.

The principle of radial keratotomy (RK) is to make deep (approximately 90% depth) radial incisions in the midperiphery of the cornea to induce central flattening and correct low degrees of myopia (typically −2.00 to −8.00D) [3, 55]. A central clear zone of about 3 mm remains untouched, and the incisions radiate from its edge towards the periphery. This generates an optical zone of about 6 mm.

Mechanisms

The radial incisions transect the collagen lamellae, thereby structurally weakening the cornea [56]. The wound gapes due to retraction of the most anterior fibres [57] and the outward force of the intraocular pressure. This causes flattening of the central cornea in the meridian of the incision and 90° away [58]. The spreading is greatest at the midpoint of the incision, (approximately at the 7-mm-diameter zone), resulting in bulging of the midperiphery (Fig. 13.2).

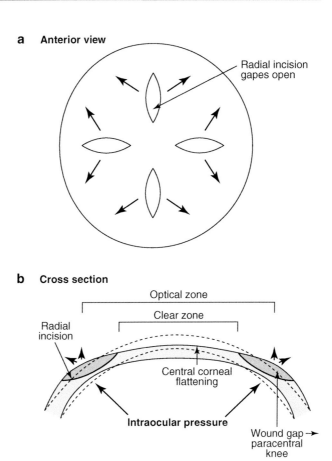

Fig. 13.2 Radial keratotomy mechanism. The radial incisions gape causing an increase in the corneal circumference, which is greatest at the midpoint of the incisions (**a**). As the limbus is fixed, the increase in circumference is accommodated by the cornea bowing forward in the midperiphery, producing a paracentral knee. This results in flattening of the central cornea (**b**)

Wound gape increases during the first week in primates (2 weeks in cats and at least 4 weeks in rabbits), as epithelium fills the incision. This is associated with progressive corneal flattening and hyperopia. Thereafter the epithelial plug is replaced with fibroblastic tissue which contracts, reducing the wound gape and returning the refraction towards emmetropia [59–61]. The "tissue addition theory" suggests that the more incisions which are made, the greater the amount of tissue that is added to the cornea, and this generates a greater refractive effect. Undercorrection usually occurs as a result of inadequate incision length or depth, whereas in overcorrection, the incisions are wide and filled with excessive epithelium and scar tissue which prevents the apposition of the wound edges.

The incisions remain as sites of weakness because epithelium can persist in the wound for at least 6 years and new collagen is deposited parallel to the wound edges rather than across the defect. They fail to demonstrate the same remodelling as seen in sutured wounds, and further widening can occur leading to long-term progressive hyperopia and instability of the refraction [62, 63].

Surgical Planning

The results of radial keratotomy for a single patient are not entirely predictable. This arises from firstly, variability of the surgical technique, and secondly, individual differences in the wound healing response. The former is minimised by utilising nomograms to determine the most appropriate surgical parameters for a given case [64].

Some topography systems include radial keratotomy planning programmes in their software (Fig. 13.3). This provides an opportunity of storing the preoperative data and accurately documenting the surgical intent (Table 13.1).

Patient Variables

All nomograms utilise the preoperative spherical equivalent refractive error in the spectacle plane, the intended correction and the age of the patient. Age is an important consideration because older patients have slower or less active healing mechanisms, and as a result a particular incision produces a greater refractive effect than it would in a younger subject. Some nomograms also include the sex of the patient and the power of their cornea (Table 13.5).

Incision Variables

Based on these parameters, a nomogram will suggest the number, length and position of the incisions required to generate the appropriate refractive change. Most surgeons use four, six or eight incisions. The first four incisions generate most of the effect of the surgery, so it is possible to perform this as a primary procedure and then

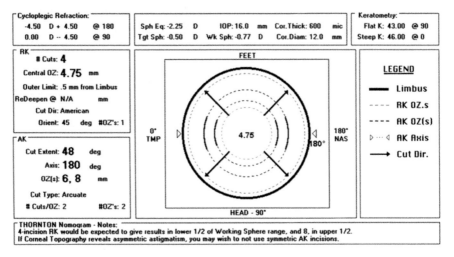

Fig. 13.3 Keratotomy planning. The site, length and depth of incisions for radial and arcuate keratotomy are determined by nomograms such as the one designed by Thornton. Having taken the topography, the surgeon enters the cycloplegic refraction (top left box) and ocular measurements (top centre box). The programme then calculates the surgical parameters for radial keratotomy (middle left box) and arcuate keratotomy (bottom left box) and displays them on a diagram (central box)

Table 13.5 The patient and surgical factors increasing the effectiveness of radial keratotomy. These variables, together with the intended refractive change, are entered into the nomograms used to plan the surgery of an individual patient

Factors increasing the effectiveness of radial keratotomy	
Patient	Increasing age
	Males
	Reduced wound healing
	Higher intraocular/atmospheric pressure
	Corneal power
Incisions	Greater number
	Longer
	Deeper
	Proximity to corneal centre
	Centripetal (Russian; as opposed to centrifugal/American)
	Inferior incisions heal more slowly

add further incisions if augmentation is required. In general 16 incisions are very rarely used at the primary procedure as this many is found to be unnecessary.

The longer and deeper the incisions are made, the greater the wound gape and the refractive effect. Initially incisions were extended out to the limbus, but nowadays shorter incisions are used with the advantages of more rapid wound healing and visual recovery, greater stability of refraction and avoidance of vascular ingrowth. In addition, central clear zones tend to be larger to prevent the glare and reduced contrast sensitivity associated with incisions overlying the pupillary aperture [63].

The direction in which the incisions are made also influences their refractive effect [63, 65]. In the American technique, incisions are made centrifugally from the paracentral area towards the limbus. A blade length set at 100% of the paracentral corneal thickness achieves an actual maximum depth of 80–85%, and this is not reached for at least the first 1 mm of the incision. The Russian technique, in which the blade is drawn centripetally, results in a deeper wound along the whole length of the incision and wider gape. This greater effect may be due to differences in the angle that the blade incises the cornea, greater efficiency in the cutting of corneal lamellae, the slower healing [62] or the fact that the exit site of a blade is wider than the entry site, and in this technique, the exit site is closest to the centre of the cornea.

Modification of Nomograms

Several nomograms are available, most of which are derived retrospectively by experts for their own-specific technique. However, when a single surgeon aims to make several identical incisions in the same cornea, with the same blade settings, the depth achieved may differ by as much as 30%. The variability between surgeons would be even greater, as relatively subtle differences in technique may have an effect, such as the instruments used, the angle of the blade, the pressure it applies to the cornea and the speed at which it is drawn through the tissues. Therefore individual surgeons need to modify the existing nomograms in the light of their own experience.

Enhancement Procedures

Enhancement procedures may be performed in as many as 20–35% of eyes undergoing radial keratotomy, and some eyes undergo three or more operations [62]. The use of a staged approach introduces a degree of adjustability which reduces the risk of overcorrection. However, it increases the time taken to achieve refractive stability, because the outcome of one procedure must be allowed to stabilise before embarking upon the next. Despite performing enhancements, the refractive results cannot be guaranteed because the nomograms are less reliable in eyes which have received previous surgery. Some patients may prefer surgical monovision in which one eye remains undercorrected to reduce symptomatic presbyopia.

Formerly enhancements were performed by reincising the original incisions, but this technique has fallen from favour because it is almost impossible to retrace exactly the original incisions. The resultant overlapping and intersection of incisions tend to lead to increased scarring.

Enhancements are usually performed by either adding four or eight incisions between the existing ones or by deepening and lengthening the primary incisions. This is performed by first opening the incisions with an intraocular lens hook and cleaning out the epithelium and then reinserting the diamond knife to extend the incision. Alternatively, additional refractive effect can be obtained by using a different refractive technique as a second procedure.

Topographic Patterns After Radial Keratotomy

Discrete radial incisions made in the midperipheral cornea result in topographic changes across the whole corneal diameter (profile) which may vary from one meridian to another (pattern) (Table 13.6). Postoperatively the corneal irregularity is greater than preoperatively, with the maximum range of dioptric powers within a 4 mm pupil increasing from 2.0D to 3.8D [63–65].

Table 13.6 The characteristic topographic changes seen after radial keratotomy

Topographic changes after radial keratotomy
Irregularity increased
Oblate profile – "negative shape factor"; corneal power decreases towards the centre
Central flattening
Peripheral steepening
Inflection zone/"paracentral knee"
Rapid change in slope between the zones of central flattening and peripheral steepening
Asphericity increased
Polygonal pattern common
Multifocal cornea range of dioptric powers within entrance pupil increased
Good visual acuity despite residual refractive error
Visual distortion despite excellent spectacle-corrected acuity

Table 13.7 Incidence of the different profiles and videokeratoscopic patterns of corneal topography after radial keratotomy, compared to normal. An oblate profile with polygonal pattern is the most common topography after radial keratotomy, but this is not seen in normal corneas

Topography		Normal [67] (%)	Radial keratotomy [66] (%)
Profile	Prolate	100	3
	Mixed prolate/oblate	0	18
	Oblate	0	79
Pattern	Round	23	6
	Oval	21	0
	Symmetric bow tie	18	16
	Asymmetric bow tie	32	6
	Irregular	7	6
	Polygonal	0	63
	Steep-flat-steep	0	34

Corneal Profile

Gaping of the radial incisions results in an annulus of corneal steepening 2.7 mm (1.75–3.3 mm) from the corneal centre. This is called the paracentral knee or inflection zone. Central to this the cornea is flattened, as required for the correction of myopia. Therefore, after RK, the corneal profile tends to be oblate, as occurs in 79% of patients, although 18% have a mixed prolate/oblate profile [66]. An oblate profile is never seen in normal corneas [67] (Table 13.7).

Postoperatively the corneal asphericity is increased, with the increase being greater in the higher magnitude corrections. In the normal cornea, the change in dioptric power from centre to periphery is −1.9D, whereas after RK, it may typically be +2.8D. The dioptric change tends to vary in different semimeridians, although it is usually greatest superiorly and inferiorly, possibly due to the pressure of the eyelid on the structurally weakened cornea [66].

Topographic Patterns

The topographic patterns resulting from RK [66] have been classified in a similar manner to those seen in normal corneas [67] (Table 13.7). After RK, four of the patterns (round, symmetric bow tie, asymmetric bow tie and irregular) were similar to those seen in normal corneas but occurred less frequently (Figs. 13.4 and 13.5). The only normal pattern not seen postoperatively was oval.

Over half (59%) of corneas which have undergone RK demonstrate a polygonal pattern, which is never seen in normal corneas (Fig. 13.6). This is a concentric pattern containing two or more angles (≤135°) and three or more nearly straight lines. The angles correspond closely with the central ends of the radial incisions, and the polygons therefore include squares, hexagons and octagons, depending upon the number of incisions. Some polygons appear incomplete or asymmetric, which may be due to variable incision lengths or depths or an improperly centred surgical procedure or topography measurement.

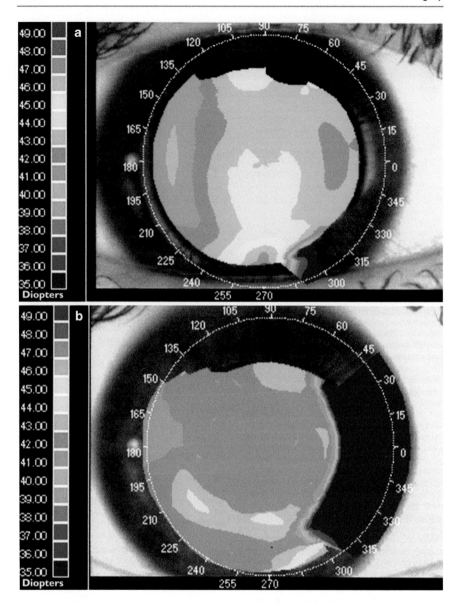

Fig. 13.4 Radial keratotomy (regular). Four-incision wide optical zone −1.00D radial keratotomy. (**a**) Preoperatively the uncorrected vision was 6/24 and the refraction −1.25D. (**b**) One month postoperatively, the central corneal power was reduced by 1.00D, the uncorrected vision was 6/5 and the optical zone had a round pattern

About half the polygons demonstrate a central nipple or steep-flat-steep pattern in which a central steep area is surrounded by an annulus of paracentral flattening and then a peripheral ring of steepening.

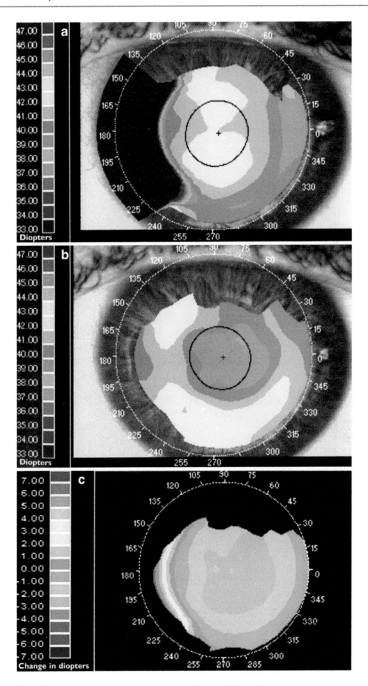

Fig. 13.5 Radial keratotomy (irregular). Four-incision −3.00D radial keratotomy plus two-incision −0.50 astigmatic keratotomy gave improvement in the uncorrected visual acuity from 6/60 to 6/6. (**a**) Preoperatively the regular bow tie showed that the cornea was steep in the vertical meridian. (**b**) One month postoperatively, the central cornea was flattened and the astigmatism corrected. The vision was good, but the topography revealed slight irregularity in the midperipheral cornea at the site of the incisions. (**c**) The difference map demonstrates the induced change in power, which is slightly greater in the vertical meridian where the astigmatic keratotomy was performed

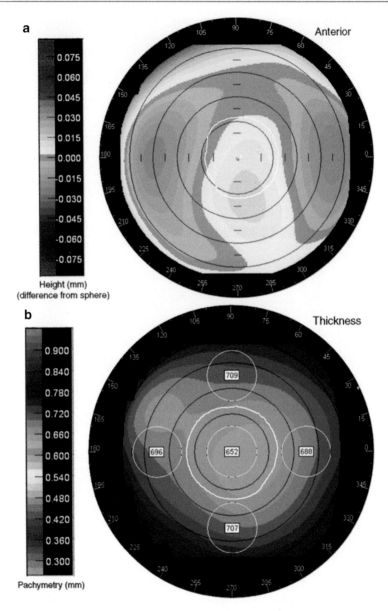

Fig. 13.6 Radial keratotomy (polygonal). A slit image system was used to assess the topography of a patient undergoing four-incision radial keratotomy. (**a**) Preoperative height of the anterior corneal surface (the reference sphere has a radius of curvature of 7.75 mm which is equivalent to 43.5D). (**b**) The corneal thickness is measured preoperatively to determine the depth to which the blade should be set. (**c**) One year postoperatively, the topography (height difference from sphere) of the anterior corneal surface was polygonal (almost square, because four incisions were made). This arose because flattening was the greatest in the meridian of the incisions, which were placed diagonally (the reference sphere has a radius of curvature of 7.97 mm which is equivalent to 42.3D)

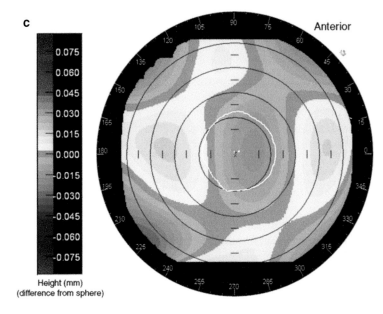

Fig. 13.6 (continued)

Eyes with least astigmatism preoperatively tend to have round or polygonal post-operative patterns. In contrast, those with greater preoperative astigmatism tend to develop a mixed prolate/oblate profile and a bow tie or irregular pattern. However postoperatively, there is no significant difference in astigmatism between the topographic patterns.

Multifocal Cornea

After RK there can be poor correlation between the residual refractive error and the measured visual acuity. This is thought to be due to the increased range of dioptric powers within the pupillary aperture enabling the cornea to act as a multifocal lens [50, 66, 68–70].

Some patients have good unaided visual acuity despite a persisting refractive error [66]. They are probably viewing light passing through a relatively small portion of cornea with a power consistent with emmetropia. However, other patients complain of visual distortion despite excellent spectacle-corrected acuity [69]. This probably arises from optical aberrations generated by light passing through adjacent portions of cornea with differing refractive powers. Under normal conditions of illumination, the paracentral knee is outside the entrance pupil and is unlikely to contribute to these effects [51].

Topographic Changes over Time After Radial Keratotomy

Maximal flattening occurs initially at the proximal end of the incisions in the para-central cornea, and the central cornea remains relatively steep. Over the following months, the flattening proceeds centripetally to include the central cornea. This may be due to a relaxation or relative sliding of severed stromal lamellae [70]. In the original studies, by 1 year, 10% of patients were overcorrected, and 30% had regressed by >1.00D [71].

Transient Central Corneal Steepening

A minority of patients develop central corneal steepening, associated with an increasingly myopic refraction, in the first day or two postoperatively [72]. This occurs when the incisions permit the entry of fluid into the stroma, causing the collagen lamellae to separate. The collagen fibres of the unincised central clear zone have a normal stress distribution which resists corneal oedema, and therefore this area stays relatively thin. An excess of midperipheral corneal oedema generates a centripetal pressure on the central clear zone, which bows forwards producing a relative steepening in this area. This situation may be associated with ocular discomfort, disruption of the epithelium and the photokeratoscopy mires over the incisions and multiple fine posterior folds perpendicular to the radial incisions.

The following day, the oedema resolves, and an exaggerated midperipheral shoulder may develop, causing excessive central flattening and overcorrection. Within a few days, this settles, leaving a final refraction close to that intended.

Diurnal Fluctuation

In a significant proportion of patients after RK, the cornea undergoes progressive steepening during the day, and this is associated with increasing myopia from morning to evening. The majority of the change occurs in the first hour after waking and is complete within a couple of hours, although in some patients, drift may continue throughout the day. These effects are greatest early after surgery and tend to reduce over time but may persist beyond 7 years [47].

Four mechanisms have been proposed to explain flattening of the incised cornea during sleep, which then reverses during the day. Firstly, although intraocular pressures above those encountered physiologically can increase wound gape [58], the 1.3–1.5 mmHg rise observed in the morning is not effective experimentally [56], and does not correlate with measured topographic or refractive changes [46, 47]. The second theory suggests a uniform increase in corneal thickness greater than the 4–8% seen in normal corneas. The measured pachymetric changes are increased in the first couple of weeks after surgery, but they are not correlated with topographic or refractive changes [46, 47]. Thirdly, variable epithelial and stromal oedema develops during sleep, and these changes in hydration may alter the stress distribution among the stromal lamellae by mechanisms similar to those described for transient corneal steepening. The in vitro hydration of a cornea which has undergone RK can cause 10D of corneal flattening [56]. Fourthly, external pressure from the closed eyelids may change the shape of the structurally weakened cornea. It is likely that visual and topographic fluctuations arise largely from a combination of the third (hydration changes) and fourth (lid pressure) mechanisms.

A diurnal refractive change of greater than 0.50D has been documented in 42% of patients at 1 year and 31% of patients at 3.5 years [23]. Subjective complaints of fluctuating vision have been found in 54% at about 1.5 years [47] and 42% at about 4 years [46] but are seldom sufficient to warrant multiple pairs of glasses. Those patients with subjective symptoms have a measured diurnal refractive change which is double that of asymptomatic patients (−0.52D versus −0.27D) [47], and their loss of visual acuity averages 2.3 lines compared to none. Undercorrected patients see better in the morning and then lose on average 3.5 lines during the day, although a maximum reduction of 8 lines has been recorded. Overcorrected patients experience improving acuity during the day, with 15% gaining more than one line [46].

Although normal corneas undergo a small amount of diurnal topographic steepening at their very centre, the effect is greater in magnitude and more widespread following RK (0.36D within 1 mm of the corneal centre versus 0.39D and 0.42D at 1 mm and 3 mm) [47]. After RK, the steepening tends to be greater inferiorly than superiorly. Several theories have been proposed to explain this, including, firstly, tension generated by the extraocular muscles during accommodative convergence and, secondly, tension in the orbicularis muscle, which has previously been suggested as a cause of inferior wound abnormalities following penetrating keratoplasty.

Visual fluctuations are more common in patients with a bow tie (dumb-bell or split optical zone) topographic pattern postoperatively. Of patients with visual fluctuations, 91% had bow tie, and 9% had round patterns. Of those without visual fluctuations, 80% had round, 20% had band-like, and none had bow tie patterns. However, it is not predictable from the preoperative topography who is likely to suffer fluctuations.

Diurnal fluctuations are more common in patients with greater than eight incisions, although they are not influenced by the length of the incisions (optical zone size) [47, 71]. Older patients tend to suffer less fluctuation than younger ones [47].

Progressive Hyperopia

Although some patients achieve stability of refraction within 6 months, a significant number have a continuing hyperopic shift for several years. In the Prospective Evaluation of Radial Keratotomy (PERK) study, 43% of patients gained more than 1.00D of hyperopia between 6 months and 10 years postoperatively [25], and there has been no evidence to suggest when this process might cease.

This instability of the corneal shape is likely to arise because the continuity of the severed collagen fibres is not restored during healing and the tensile strength of the lamellae is consequently permanently reduced [73].

No patient variable such as age or intraocular pressure has been found to be associated with biomechanical, topographic or refractive instability, and the effects of atmospheric pressure are not well understood. However, it is thought that progressive hyperopia is more common following incisions which are deeper or longer (central clear zone of 3.0 mm compared to 3.5 or 4.0 mm). Mini-RK is a modified procedure which tries to overcome this instability by using shorter incisions, as it is the paracentral part of the incision which creates most of the refractive effect. Alternatively, some surgeons intentionally undercorrect patients by 0.50–1.00D to delay the onset of hyperopia.

Long-Term Instability
Progressive hyperopia is the commonest form of long-term instability, but a minority of patients experience continuing loss of refractive effect/regression (4%) or fluctuation without a definite trend (14%) [25]. Changes in intraocular pressure have no effect within the normal range, but altitude (reduced atmospheric pressure) can be associated with corneal flattening years after the topography has been otherwise stable [56].

Astigmatic Keratotomy

Astigmatism is the refractive error in which light is not focused at a single point, owing to the unequal refraction of light in different meridians (Chap. 6). Regular astigmatism is where the refractive power changes gradually from one meridian to the next in uniform increments, resulting in an optical system with the axes of the greatest and least power being perpendicular, and results in a focal line. Such a defect is correctable by a spherocylindrical lens, whereas irregular astigmatism is not. Regular astigmatism may be naturally occurring or surgically induced by procedures such as cataract extraction or keratoplasty [74]. It can be corrected by incisional procedures, or if a patient is undergoing cataract surgery, a toric IOL can be considered if the astigmatism is stable [75].

Mechanisms

Regular astigmatism is potentially correctable by a variety of corneal procedures, which fall into two main groups: those which flatten the steep meridian and those which steepen the flat meridian. In both cases, the induced change in the operated meridian is associated with the reverse change in the perpendicular meridian, in a process called "coupling" (Fig. 9.1).

Coupling is likely to result from the presence of intact rings of collagen lamellae running circumferentially around the base of the cornea. As a result of surgery in the operated meridian, these rings become oval and thereby transmit forces to the unoperated meridian.

The "coupling ratio" compares the dioptric flattening in one meridian to the dioptric steepening in the perpendicular meridian. If the flattening and steepening are of the same magnitude, the coupling ratio is 1:1, and there should be no net change in the spherical equivalent. If there is excessive flattening compared to steepening (e.g. a ratio of 2:1 is not uncommon), there will be an associated hyperopic shift in the spherical equivalent.

Compressive Procedures
Wedge resection and compressive sutures can each be performed alone or in combination. Both aim to steepen the flat meridian by depressing the limbal cornea [76] (Fig. 11.1a). Therefore the excision of tissue or the row of tight sutures is centred on the flat meridian in the periphery and may be paired with a similar procedure performed 180° away. These techniques are mainly useful for the very

high degrees of astigmatism (e.g. >12.00 DC) induced by surgery and may be combined with wound revision [75].

Relaxing Procedures

Relaxing procedures are centred over the steep meridian with the aim of causing flattening. The technique which is easiest to perform is the release of tight sutures in the steep meridian following corneal surgery (Figs. 11.1a, 11.5 and 12.5).

The remaining techniques involve placing corneal incisions peripherally in the steep meridian with the aim of producing wound gape. This steepens the cornea immediately overlying the incision and flattens the cornea central to it (Fig. 13.7). If performed singly, flattening is also achieved in the axis 180° away. However, the procedures are most commonly paired, in which case they are performed at both ends of the steep meridian.

Fig. 13.7 Arcuate keratotomy mechanism. Circumferential incisions are centred on the steep axis and are frequently paired (**a**). Gaping of the wound causes peripheral bowing with local steepening and central flattening in that meridian (**b**). The intact collagen lamellae around the base of the cornea are stretched and become oval. These forces are transmitted to the perpendicular meridian where they cause central steepening as a result of coupling (**c**)

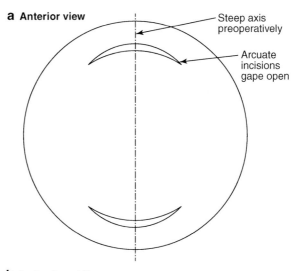

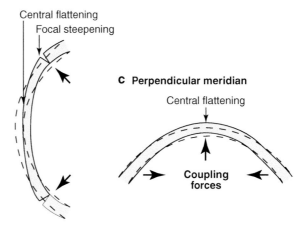

Coupling results in steepening of the perpendicular flat meridian. The astigmatic change achieved is the sum of the flattening in one axis and the steepening in the perpendicular axis. However, when results are analysed and presented, they should be expressed as the "vector-corrected change in astigmatism" which takes account of the change in the axis of the astigmatism as well as its magnitude [77–81].

The incisional techniques used initially were developed from radial keratotomy but applied in a localised manner so that the flattening affected only one meridian. Initially a series of peripheral incisions were placed parallel to the steep meridian [68]. It was then realised that a greater effect could be achieved by placing incisions across the steep meridian, so that the wound gape produced a maximal increase in the radius of curvature in the required direction. Trapezoidal keratotomy was a combination of parallel and transverse incisions in the steep axis but was associated with corneal scarring and irregularity and a large hyperopic shift. These complications were greater if the incisions intersected [77].

Relaxing incisions have been largely superseded by laser corrective procedures. If performed, they are placed solely across the steep meridian. In transverse keratotomy (T-cuts), the incisions are straight and are relatively easily performed freehand with a guarded blade or diamond knife [82]. In arcuate keratotomy (circumferential relaxing incisions), the incisions are curved parallel to the limbus. This technique is facilitated by the use of semiautomated devices such as the Hanna arcuate keratome [83].

Surgical Planning

The outcome of astigmatic keratotomy is affected by similar variables to those influencing radial keratotomy, and likewise, the results are not entirely predictable. Nomograms have been developed to suggest the number, length, depth and position of the incisions required to generate the appropriate refractive change [82, 84], and these have been included in topographic software (Fig. 13.8).

Transverse keratotomy incisions are usually 1–4 mm long, 80–90% of the corneal thickness and placed at the 5–8 mm optical zones [82]. If greater effect is required, a second pair of incisions can be added 2 mm peripheral to the first.

Arcuate keratotomy, although more difficult to perform, has several advantages over transverse keratotomy. Firstly, the entire incision length is equidistant from the corneal centre. Therefore the blade encounters a similar thickness of cornea throughout the incision (apart from the nasal/temporal disparity), and the effects may be more regular. Secondly, the incision length can be measured in degrees or clock hours rather than millimetres, and therefore its effectiveness is not dependent upon its proximity to the corneal centre. Thirdly, the incisions can be of any length as they are not limited by encountering the limbus.

Arcuate keratotomies are usually one to three clock hours, performed at one third to two-thirds of the corneal depth [83–86]. Maximal effect can be achieved by paired incisions of four clock hours, although this can result in large topographic changes and excessive wound gape.

After corneal graft surgery, the results are less predictable than in normal corneas because of altered biomechanics, scarring at the donor-recipient interface, and possibly the underlying disease [87]. Most surgeons prefer arcuate keratotomies in the graft rather than opening the graft-host (donor-recipient) junction because there is better control of the surgery, less risk of leakage or dehiscence and more consistent wound healing [85]. In cases of asymmetric astigmatism, asymmetric length and placement of incisions has been advocated [76, 83].

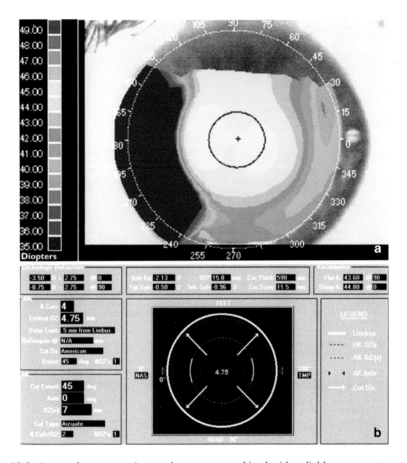

Fig. 13.8 Arcuate keratotomy. Arcuate keratotomy combined with radial keratotomy to correct −0.75/−2.75 ×90° in the left eye. (**a**) Preoperatively there was a horizontal steep bow tie consistent with against-the-rule astigmatism (tangential maps). (**b**) The refraction was entered in the top left box and the other corneal parameters in the top centre box. The keratometry from the preoperative map appears in the top right box. According to the Thornton nomogram, the software suggested that for the radial keratotomy (middle left box), four cuts be made centrifugally (American-style) from a 4.75 mm optical to within 0.5 mm of the limbus. It also suggested that two arcuate incisions (bottom left box) of length 45° should be made at the 7 mm optical zone, centred on 0° meridian. The surgical plan is shown diagrammatically in the central box, with a key to the right. (**c**) One month postoperatively, the refraction was −0.75DS, and the tangential topography map showed regular central flattening with loss of the bow tie pattern. However, there was local steepening, particularly temporally but also nasally, due to the midperipheral bulging associated with the incisions. (**d**) The difference map demonstrates how the arcuate incisions have achieved flattening in the horizontal axis. This was associated with slight steepening in the vertical axis as a result of coupling, but the effect was less marked due to the low-dioptre radial keratotomy procedure performed simultaneously, which slightly flattened the whole cornea

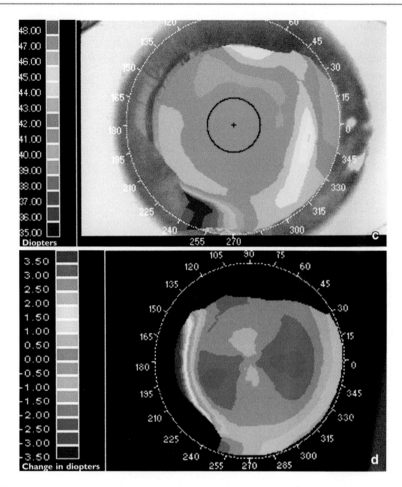

Fig. 13.8 (continued)

Some surgeons combine astigmatic procedures with spherical refractive surgery or cataract extraction [88, 89] (Fig. 13.8), whilst others believe that a staged approach is preferable. Astigmatism can unintentionally be altered by spherical procedures, so it may be more accurate to delay astigmatic surgery until after the refraction has stabilised (Fig. 13.5).

Topography After Astigmatic Keratotomy

Preoperatively the topography of the majority of corneas has a bow tie configuration (Fig. 13.8), and in most, it is asymmetric, particularly following previous corneal surgery.

Relaxing incisions induce flattening of the steep meridian, and usually an equal or slightly lesser steepening of the perpendicular meridian, depending upon the coupling ratio. Localised peripheral steepening over the incision itself may be visible on some maps. The topography usually stabilises by 8 weeks postoperatively. Most procedures are about 70% effective in reducing astigmatism, although they may be associated with a change in axis of about 20°.

For arcuate keratotomies, the most common postoperative topographic pattern is a bow tie with rounded ends, which may be symmetric or asymmetric [86]. Transverse keratotomies more frequently generate a bow tie with flattened ends, or polygonal or irregular patterns, which resemble the shape of the incisions made on the surface of the cornea. This may be because the depth and the proximity to the corneal centre vary along the length of the incision.

Polygonal and irregular patterns are more commonly seen following trapezoidal than arcuate keratotomy and in corneas following keratoplasty than in those with naturally occurring astigmatism [77]. This may result from loss of the normal biomechanical properties of the cornea due to transection of more collagen lamellae and scarring at the graft-host interface in cases of keratoplasty (Chap. 11). These factors may also limit the amount of coupling which can occur and therefore account for the higher flattening/steepening coupling ratios seen in these two groups. They also demonstrate a greater range of dioptric powers within the pupil margin, which is responsible for the glare and visual distortion experienced.

Intrastromal Corneal Rings

Intrastromal corneal rings modify the corneal shape by altering the stress equilibria in the collagen lamellae. However, they achieve this by applying pressure and taking up space, rather than dividing them in the manner performed in incisional refractive surgery. Therefore the major advantage of intrastromal rings over incisional procedures is that they are reversible and the cornea returns to approximately its former shape when the rings are removed.

A ring is composed of optically transparent polymethylmethacrylate and takes the form of a complete 360° circle with a single break or two 150° segments (Fig. 13.9). The device is inserted through a 1.8–2.0 mm peripheral radial incision at 12 o'clock and fed into a predissected circumferential channel at two-thirds of the stromal depth. The minimum central optical zone is 7 mm.

Mechanisms

It was initially thought that intrastromal rings would correct myopia by applying a centrifugal force to the periphery of the cornea and thereby flattened the centre. However, it is now considered that the ring acts as a spacer and that by separating the corneal lamellae so they pass around the upper or lower surface of the ring, it shortens their effective arc from limbus to limbus (Fig. 13.10). The thickness of the device is linearly related to the degree of flattening induced. Rings ranging from 0.25 to 0.45 mm in thickness correct myopia of −1.00 to −5.00D [90]. Pairs of ring

Fig. 13.9 Intrastromal corneal ring (photograph). An intrastromal corneal ring composed of two segments

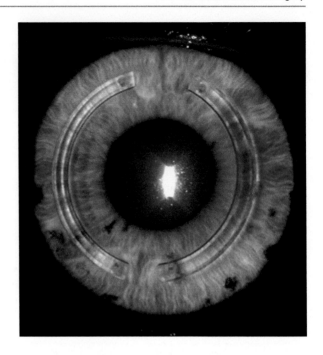

Fig. 13.10 Intrastromal corneal ring mechanism. The ring is inserted at two-thirds depth in the peripheral cornea. It increases the arc length of the collagen fibres and thereby flattens the central cornea

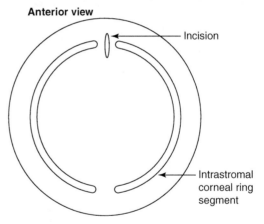

segments of differing thicknesses have been used to address irregular astigmatism. In some cases of keratoconus, a single ring segment has been used in the sector of maximal steepening.

Topography After Intrastromal Corneal Rings

The insertion of intrastromal rings has an immediate topographic effect which reverses when the rings are removed. The ring itself is evident as a peripheral annulus of local steepening, within which the central cornea is flattened (Fig. 13.11). This technique has the advantage over many other refractive procedures that the natural aspheric prolate shape of the central cornea is relatively maintained.

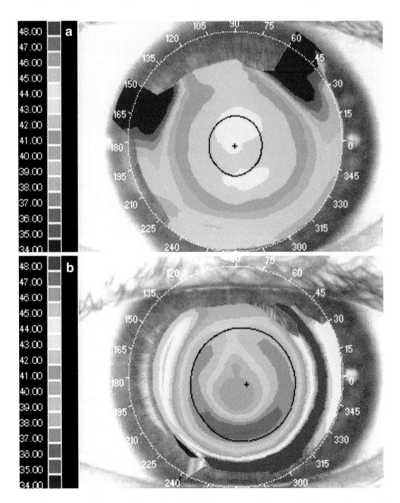

Fig. 13.11 Intrastromal corneal ring. A −2.50D intrastromal corneal ring was inserted as two segments. (**a**) Preoperatively the topography was normal with minimal with-the-rule astigmatism (tangential maps). (**b**) Three months postoperatively, the central cornea was flattened, and there was an annulus of steepening in the periphery associated with the ring. (**c**) The difference map demonstrates the change achieved by the surgery. This is reversible upon removal of the rings

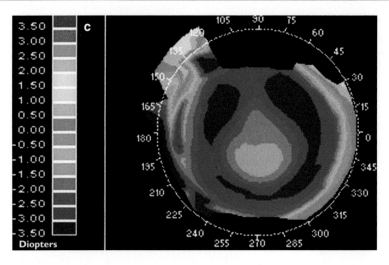

Fig. 13.11   (continued)

References

References Particularly Worth Reading

1. Waring GO. Development and evaluation of refractive surgical procedures. Part I. Five stages in the continuum of development. J Refract Surg. 1987;3:141–57.
2. Javitt JC. Clear lens extraction for high myopia: is this an idea whose time has come? [editorial]. Arch Ophthalmol. 1994;112:321–3.
3. Rosen ES. Considering corneal and lenticular techniques of refractive surgery [editorial]. J Cat Refract Surg. 1997;23:689–91.
4. Maguire LJ. Corneal topography of patients with excellent Snellen visual acuity after epikeratophakia for aphakia. Am J Ophthalmol. 1990;109:162–7.
5. Li SM, Kang MT, Zhou Y, et al. Wavefront excimer laser refractive surgery for adults with refractive errors. Cochrane Database Syst Rev. 2017;6:CD012687.
6. Moreira H, Campos M, Sawusch MR, et al. Holmium laser thermokeratoplasty. Ophthalmology. 1993;100(5):752–61.
7. Thornton SP. Clinical evaluation of corneal topography. J Cat Refract Surg. 1993;19(Suppl):198–202.
8. Young JA, Kornmehl EW. Chapter 16 – Preoperative evaluation for refractive surgery. Posted on medtextfree on November 12, 2010 in Ophthalmology. n.d..
9. Ambrósio R Jr, Klyce SD, Wilson SE. Corneal topographic and pachymetric screening of keratorefractive patients. J Refract Surg. 2003;19:24–9.
10. *Wilson SE, Klyce SD. Screening for corneal topographic abnormalities before refractive surgery. Ophthalmology. 1994;101:147–52.
11. Nesburn AB, Bahri S, Salz J, Rabinowitz YS, Maguen E, Hofbauer J, Belin M, Macy JI. Keratoconus detected by videokeratography in candidates for photorefractive keratectomy. J Refract Surg. 1995;11:194–201.
12. Bowman CB, Thompson KP, Stulting RD. Refractive keratotomy in keratoconus suspects. J Refract Surg. 1995;11:202–6.
13. Doyle SJ, Hynes E, Naroo S, Shah S. PRK in patients with a keratoconic topography picture. The concept of a physiological 'displaced apex syndrome'. Br J Ophthalmol. 1996;80:25–8.

14. Colin J, Cochener B, Bobo C, Malet F, Gallinaro C, Le Floch G. Myopic photorefractive keratectomy in eyes with atypical inferior corneal steepening. J Cataract Refract Surg. 1996;22:1423–6.
15. Wilson SE, Lin DTC, Klyce SD, Reidy JJ, Insler MS. Topographic changes in contact lens-induced warpage. Ophthalmology. 1990;97:734–44.
16. Ruiz-Montenegro J, Mafra CH, Wilson SE, Jumper JM, Klyce SD, Mendelson EN. Corneal topographic alterations in normal contact lens wearers. Ophthalmology. 1993;100:128–34.
17. Corbett MC, O'Brart DPS, Marshall J. Biological and environmental risk factors for regression after photorefractive keratectomy. Ophthalmology. 1996;103:1381–91.
18. Lebow KA, Grohe R. Differentiating contact lens induced warpage from true keratoconus using corneal topography. Eye Contact Lens. 1999;25:114.
19. Randleman JB, Woodward M, Lynn MJ, et al. Risk assessment of ectasia after corneal refractive surgery. Ophthalmology. 2008;115:37–50.
20. Santhiago MR, et al. Association between the percent tissue altered and post–laser in situ keratomileusis ectasia in eyes with normal preoperative topography. Am J Ophthalmol. 2014;158(1):87–95.
21. Lui Z, Pflugfelder SC. Corneal surface regularity and the effect of artificial tears in aqueous tear deficiency. Ophthalmology. 1999;106(5):939–43.
22. Lui Z, Pflugfelder SC. The effects of long-term contact lens wear on corneal thickness, curvature, and surface regularity. Ophthalmology. 2000;107(1):105–11.
23. Maguire LJ, Klyce SD, Sawelson H, McDonald MB, Kaufman HE. Visual distorsion after myopic keratomileusis. Computer analysis of keratoscope photographs. Ophthalmic Surg. 1987;18:352–6.
24. Rashid ER, Waring GO. Complications of radial and transverse keratotomy. Surv Ophthalmol. 1989;34:74–104.
25. *Waring GO III, Lynn MJ, McDonnell PJ, the PERK Study Group. Results of the prospective evaluation of radial keratotomy (PERK) study ten years after surgery. Ophthalmology. 1994;112:1298–308.
26. McDonnell PJ, Caroline PJ, Salz J. Irregular astigmatism after radial and astigmatic keratotomy. Am J Ophthalmol. 1989;107:42–6.
27. *Astin CLK, Gartry DS, Steele ADMcG. Contact lens fitting after photorefractive keratectomy. Br J Ophthalmol. 1996;80:597–603.
28. Siganos DS, Pallikaris IG, Lambropoulos JE, Koufala CJ. Keratometric readings after photorefractive keratectomy are unreliable for calculating IOL power. J Refract Surg. 1996;12:S278–9.
29. Pepose JS, Lim-Bon-Siong R, Mardelli P. Future shock: the long term consequences of refractive surgery. Br J Ophthalmol. 1997;81:428–9.
30. Lesher MP, Schumer DJ, Hunkeler JD, Durrie DS, McKee FE. Phacoemulsification with intraocular lens implantation after excimer photorefractive keratectomy: a case report. J Cataract Refract Surg. 1994;20(Suppl):265–7.
31. Hoffer KJ. Calculating intraocular lens power after refractive corneal surgery [editorial]. Arch Ophthalmol. 2002;120:500–1.
32. Koch DD, Wang L. Calculating IOL power in eyes that have had refractive surgery. J Cataract Refract Surg. 2003;29:2039–42.
33. Savini G, Hoffer KJ, Zanini M. IOL power calculations after LASIK and PRK. Cataract Refract Surg Today Eur. 2007;4:37–44.
34. Feiz V, Mannis MJ. Intraocular lens calculations after corneal refractive surgery. Curr Opin Ophthalmol. 2004;15:342–9.
35. Hodge C, McAlinden C, Lawless M, et al. Intraocular lens power calculation following laser refractive surgery. Eye Vision. 2015;2:7.
36. Klyce SD, Smolek MK. Corneal topography of excimer laser photorefractive keratectomy. J Cataract Refract Surg. 1993;19(Suppl):122–30.
37. Uozato H, Guyton DL. Centering corneal surgical procedures. Am J Ophthalmol. 1987;103:264–75.

38. Guyton DL. More on optical zone centration [letter]. Ophthalmology. 1994;101:793.
39. Fleming JF. Should refractive surgeons worry about corneal asphericity? Refract Corneal Surg. 1990;6:455–7.
40. Eghbali F, Yeung KK, Maloney RK. Topographic determination of corneal asphericity and its lack of effect on the outcome of radial keratotomy. Am J Ophthalmol. 1995;119:275–80.
41. Seiler T, Reckmann W, Maloney RK. Effective spherical aberration of the cornea as a quantitative descriptor in corneal topography. J Cataract Refract Surg. 1993;19(Suppl):155–65.
42. Oliver KM, Hemenger RP, Corbett MC, O'Brart DPS, Verma S, Marshall J, Tomlinson A. Corneal optical aberrations induced by photorefractive keratectomy. J Refract Surg. 1997;13:246–54.
43. Maguire LJ, Zabel RW, Parker P, Lindstrom RL. Topography and raytracing analysis of patients with excellent visual acuity 3 months after excimer laser photorefractive keratectomy for myopia. Refract Corneal Surg. 1991;7:122–8.
44. Schwartz-Goldstein BH, Hersh PS, The Summit Photorefractive Keratectomy Topography Study Group. Corneal topography of phase III excimer laser photorefractive keratectomy: optical zone centration analysis. Ophthalmology. 1995;102:951–62.
45. Cantera E, Cantera I, Olivieri L. Corneal topographic analysis of photorefractive keratectomy in 175 myopic eyes. Refract Corneal Surg. 1993;9(Suppl):S19–22.
46. *McDonnell PJ, McClusky DJ, Garbus J. Corneal topography and fluctuating visual acuity after radial keratotomy. Ophthalmology. 1989;96:665–70.
47. *Kwitko S, Gritz DC, Garbus JJ, Gauderman WJ, McDonnell PJ. Diurnal variation of corneal topography after radial keratotomy. Arch Ophthalmol. 1992;110:351–6.
48. Lin DTC. Corneal topographic analysis after excimer laser photorefractive keratectomy. Ophthalmology. 1994;101:1423–39.
49. Moreno-Barrusio E, Merayo Lloves J, Marcos S, et al. Ocular aberrations before and after myopic corneal refractive surgery: LASIK-induced changes measured with laser ray tracing. IOVS. 2001;42:1396–403.
50. Holladay JT, Lumm MJ, Waring GO III, Gemmil M, Keehn GC, Fielding B. The relationship of visual acuity, refractive error; and pupil size after radial keratotomy. Arch Ophthalmol. 1991;109:70–6.
51. Applegate RA, Gansel KA. The importance of pupil size in optical quality measurements following radial keratotomy. Refract Corneal Surg. 1990;6:47–54.
52. Binder PS. Optical problems following refractive surgery. Ophthalmology. 1986;93:739–45.
53. Balakrishnan V, Lim ASM, Tseng PSF, Hong LC. Decentered ablation zones resulting from photorefractive keratectomy with an erodible mask. Int Ophthalmol. 1993;17:179–84.
54. McDonnell JP, Garbus FG. Corneal topographic changes after radial keratotomy. Refract Corneal Surg. 1989;5:379–87.
55. Fyodorov SN, Durnev VA. Surgical correction of complicated myopic astigmatism by means of dissection of the circular ligament of the cornea. Ann Ophthalmol. 1981;13:115.
56. Simon G, Ren Q. Biomechanical behaviour of the cornea and its response to radial keratotomy. J Refract Corneal Surg. 1994;10:343–56.
57. Seiler T, Matallana M, Sendler S, Bende T. Does Bowman's layer determine the biomechanical properties of the cornea? Refract Corneal Surg. 1992;8:139–42.
58. Buzard KA, Ronk JF, Friedlander MH, Tepper DJ, Hoeltzel DA, Choe K-I. Quantitative measurement of wound spreading in radial keratotomy. Refract Corneal Surg. 1992;8:217–23.
59. Jester JV, Petroll WM, Feng W, Essepian J, Cavanagh HD. Radial keratotomy: the wound healing process and measurement of incisional gape in two animal models using in vivo confocal microscopy. Invest Ophthalmol Vis Sci. 1992;33:3255–70.
60. Garana RMR, Petroll M, Chen WT, Herman IM, Barry P, Andrews P, Cavanagh HD, Jester JV. Radial keratotomy: role of the myofibroblast in corneal wound contraction. Invest Ophthalmol Vis Sci. 1992;33:3271–82.
61. Petroll WM, New K, Sachdev M, Cavanagh HD, Jester JV. Radial keratotomy: relationship between wound gape and corneal curvature in primate eyes. Invest Ophthalmol Vis Sci. 1992;33:3283–91.

62. Binder PS. What we have learned about corneal wound healing from refractive surgery. Refract Corneal Surg. 1989;5:98–120.
63. Melles GR, Binder PS, Anderson JA. Variation in healing throughout the depth of long-term, unsutured, corneal wounds in human autopsy specimens and monkeys. Arch Ophthalmol. 1994;112:100–9.
64. Thornton S. A computerised nomogram for the performance of radial and arcuate keratotomy. USA: EyeSys Co; 1993.
65. Melles GRJ, Binder PS. Effect of wound location, orientation, direction, and postoperative time on unsutured corneal wound healing morphology in monkeys. Refract Corneal Surg. 1992;8:427–38.
66. *Bogan S, Maloney R, Drews C, Waring GO III. Computer-assisted videokeratography of corneal topography after radial keratotomy. Arch Ophthalmol. 1991;109:834–41.
67. Bogan SJ, Waring GO, Ibrahim O, Drews C, Curtis L. Classification of normal corneal topography based on computer-assisted videokeratography. Arch Ophthalmol. 1990;108:945–9.
68. *McDonnell PJ, Garbus J. Corneal topographic changes after radial keratotomy. Ophthalmology. 1989;96:45–9.
69. Maguire LJ, Bourne WM. A multifocal lens effect as a complication of radial keratotomy. J Refract Corneal Surg. 1989;5:394–9.
70. *Moreira H, Fasano AP, Garbus JJ, Lee M, McDonnell PJ. Corneal topographic changes over time after radial keratotomy. Cornea. 1992;11:465–70.
71. Waring GO III, Lynn M, Gelender H, Laibson P, Lindstrom R, Myers W, the PERK Study Group. Results of the prospective evaluation of radial keratotomy (PERK) study one year after surgery. Ophthalmology. 1985;92:177–98.
72. *Buzard KA, Fundingsland BR, Friedlander M. Transient central corneal steepening after radial keratotomy. J Refract Surg. 1996;12:521–5.
73. Buzard KA. Introduction to biomechanics of the cornea [review]. Refract Corneal Surg. 1992;8:126–38.
74. *Swinger CA. Postoperative astigmatism. Surv Ophthalmol. 1987;31:219–48.
75. Kessel L, Andresen J, Tendal B, et al. Toric intraocular lenses in the correction of astigmatism during cataract surgery: a systematic review and meta-analysis. Ophthalmology. 2016;123(2):275–86.
76. *van Rij G, Waring GO III. Changes in corneal curvature induced by sutures and incisions. Am J Ophthalmol. 1984;98:773–83.
77. *Harto MA, Maldononado MJ, Cisneros AL, Perez-Torregrosa VT, Menezo JL. Comparison of intersecting trapezoidal keratotomy and arcuate transverse keratotomy in the correction of high astigmatism. J Refract Surg. 1996;12:585–94.
78. Calossi A, Verzella F, Penso A. Computer program to calculate vectorial change of refraction induced by refractive surgery. Refract Corneal Surg. 1993;9:276–9.
79. Vass C, Menapace R. Computerised statistical analysis of corneal topography for the evaluation of changes in corneal shape after surgery. Am J Ophthalmol. 1994;118:177–84.
80. Olsen T, Dam-Johansen M, Beke T, Hjortdal JO. Evaluating surgically induced astigmatism by Fourier analysis of corneal topography data. J Cataract Refract Surg. 1996;22:318–23.
81. Alpins NA. New method of targeting vectors to treat astigmatism. J Cataract Refract Surg. 1997;23:65–75.
82. *Güell JL, Manero F, Müller A. Transverse keratotomy to correct high corneal astigmatism after cataract surgery. J Cataract Refract Surg. 1996;22:331–6.
83. Pallikaris IG, Xirafis ME, Naoumidis LP, Siganos DS. Arcuate transverse keratotomy with a mechanical arcutome based on videokeratography. J Refract Surg. 1996;12:S296–9.
84. *Lundergan MK, Rowsey JJ. Relaxing incisions: corneal topography. Ophthalmology. 1985;92:1226–36.
85. *Duffy RJ Jain VN, Tchah H, Hofmann RF, Lindstrom RL. Paired arcuate keratotomy: a surgical approach to mixed myopic astigmatism. Arch Ophthalmol. 1988;106:1130–5.
86. McCluskey DJ, Villasenor R, McDonnell PJ. Prospective topographic analysis in peripheral arcuate keratotomy for astigmatism. Ophthalmic Surg. 1990;21:464–71.

87. Troutman RC, Swinger CA. Relaxing incision for control of postoperative astigmatism follow-
    ing keratoplasty. Ophthalmic Surg. 1980;90:131–6.
88. Ring CP, Hadden OB, Morris AT. Transverse keratotomy combined with spherical pho-
    torefractive keratectomy for compound myopic astigmatism. J Refract Corneal Surg.
    1994;10(Suppl):217–21.
89. Hall GW, Campion M, Sorenson CM, Monthofer S. Reduction of corneal astigmatism at cata-
    ract surgery. J Cataract Refract Surg. 1991;17:407–14.
90. *Schanzlin DJ, Asbell PA, Burris TE, Durrie DS. Intrastromal corneal ring segments: phase II
    results for the correction of myopia. Ophthalmology. 1997;104:1067–78.

Refractive Laser Surgery

14

Corneal refractive surgery is effective through one of two mechanisms: firstly by altering the shape of the whole thickness of the corneal stroma (Chap. 13) or secondly by affecting only the anterior corneal surface (*this chapter*).

Mechanisms

The aims of superficial procedures are the same as those of full-thickness procedures: the central cornea is flattened to correct myopia, steepened to correct hyperopia and altered in the appropriate meridian for astigmatism (Chap. 13).

In superficial procedures, tissue is either added to the anterior corneal surface (e.g. epikeratophakia [1]), removed (e.g. keratectomy and excimer or femtosecond laser procedures) or structurally altered (laser thermokeratoplasty). Of those procedures removing tissue, photorefractive keratectomy (PRK) removes tissue from the corneal surface, whereas laser in situ keratomileusis (LASIK) and femtosecond small incision lenticule extraction (SMILE) remove tissue from just below the surface, under a flap or within the anterior stroma. All these superficial techniques, unlike incisional refractive surgery or intrastromal rings, maintain the integrity of the deep corneal stroma, and the shape of the posterior corneal surface remains unaltered.

Topography for Superficial Procedures

The role of topography is similar for all forms of refractive surgery (Tables 13.1 and 13.2). The value of the topographic information obtained can be enhanced by using facilities such as the local radius of curvature, difference maps and statistical indices.

However, one limitation of topography after superficial procedures is that there is an error (about 11.4% for PRK) in the absolute corneal power reading [2]. This is

© Springer Nature Switzerland AG 2019
M. Corbett et al., *Corneal Topography*,
https://doi.org/10.1007/978-3-030-10696-6_14

because the shape of the anterior corneal surface is changed by the procedure, without the corresponding change occurring in the posterior surface. Topography systems use the standardised keratometry index (SKI) to convert measurements of radius of curvature of the anterior corneal surface into estimates of total corneal power (Table 1.1). This value is an estimate and makes an assumption about the power of the posterior corneal surface based on the measured anterior surface and knowledge of the normal corneal thickness, which is no longer applicable after surgery.

Photorefractive Keratectomy

All refractive procedures have, to some extent, suboptimal accuracy, predictability and stability of the refractive change and adverse effects on the quality of vision [3]. These shortcomings arise from two sources: firstly, the variations and inaccuracies inherent within the surgical techniques and, secondly, individual differences in the wound healing response. The first of these problems is a major contributor to the variability of the outcome of incisional procedures. However, this aspect has been largely overcome by the use of the excimer and, more recently, the femtosecond lasers in refractive surgery.

Mechanism

Excimer Laser

The excimer laser was introduced into ophthalmology in the early 1980s, when it was realised that it had characteristics ideally suited to performing refractive surgery [4, 5]. This laser could remove tissue with submicron precision, leaving a smooth surface with minimal damage to adjacent structures [6, 7]. When the beam was configured as a narrow slit, it could be used as an efficient scalpel blade to incise corneal tissue [8, 9]. However, the ability of the laser to generate a broad beam provided the additional benefit of being able to remove tissue from relatively large areas [5]. Using this technique, it became possible to change the power of the cornea by the differential ablation of superficial tissue to change its anterior curvature (photorefractive keratectomy, PRK). This avoided the weakening of the globe associated with other popular refractive procedures of the time, such as radial keratotomy.

The term "excimer" is a contraction of the words "excited dimer". Excited dimers are two atoms of an inert gas bound in a highly excited state with atoms of halogen. The excimer lasers used for refractive surgery contain argon fluoride. The decay one of these unstable molecules is accompanied by the emission of a highly energetic photon of light in the far ultraviolet portion of the spectrum (UVC, 193 nm). Each individual photon has sufficient energy to break a covalent bond, by the process termed photoablation. When this occurs in biological tissues, the cleaved macro-molecule rapidly expands and is ejected from the surface at high speed [5].

Ultraviolet C radiation has a penetration depth of less than 1 μm. Each photon emitted is absorbed by a single molecule, and therefore adjacent areas beyond 60–200 nm show no conductive effect. Each pulse removes a well-defined layer of corneal stroma 0.25 μm thick, leaving the underlying tissue undisturbed. The ablated surface is smooth and is immediately sealed by a pseudomembrane [6]. This is a layer 20–100 nm thick formed by the random recombination of double bonds uncoupled during the ablation process.

Wound Healing

In photorefractive keratectomy (PRK), the corneal epithelium is first removed, and then the excimer laser is used to ablate the underlying stroma. During the subsequent healing period, the wound is resurfaced by epithelium in a few days, and then new subepithelial tissue is produced and remodelled in a process taking many months [10–12]. The corresponding refractive changes comprise an initial overcorrection, followed by a gradual reduction in refractive error until a plateau is reached near emmetropia (or the intended refraction).

The variability of the refractive outcome after PRK arises from individual differences in the wound healing response. All patients can be considered to lie on a spectrum of wound healing [13]. The majority are near the centre, with normal healing resulting in approximately emmetropia. At one end of the spectrum are those patients with a limited healing response, who remain overcorrected with a relatively large change in corneal topography. At the other end of the spectrum are those with an aggressive healing response, who regress with a return towards their original refraction. Similarly, the topography reverts towards normal, with the treatment zone becoming much less obvious.

Myopia

To correct myopia, the excimer laser flattens the central cornea by etching a negative lens into its anterior surface (Figs. 14.1, 14.2 and 14.3). This may be achieved by passing a broad beam of relatively uniform energy distribution through either an expanding aperture, a preshaped erodible mask or a rotating slit [14]. As a result, a greater number of pulses fall on the centre than the periphery of the treatment zone, and a saucer-shaped disc of tissue is removed. The computer-controlled expansion of the aperture, the shape of the mask or slit or the movement of a flying spot determines the exact profile of the ablation. The depth of ablation is greater for corrections of higher magnitudes and larger diameters. However, still only the very superficial corneal layers are removed; for example, a −6.00D 6 mm correction has a central ablation depth of 78 μm [15].

Hyperopia

The correction of hyperopia requires the optical zone to be steepened (Fig. 14.4). This is achieved by removing an annulus of tissue from the midperiphery of the cornea [16, 17]. Therefore ablation zones need to be much larger than for the correction of myopia and are typically about 9 mm in diameter.

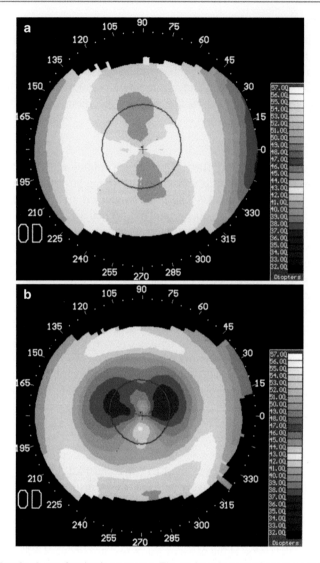

Fig. 14.1 Myopic photorefractive keratectomy. The excimer laser removes more tissue from the centre than the periphery of the treatment zone to correct myopia. This patient underwent a spherical −6.00D 6 mm PRK. (**a**) Preoperatively there was −2.00D with-the-rule astigmatism. (**b**) At 1 week postoperatively, the majority of patients are overcorrected, and in this case, the spherical equivalent was +1.50D. The contours are closest together just inside the edge of the treatment zone. There was marked flattening of the central cornea making the cornea oblate rather than prolate. Therefore the astigmatism appeared as a blue horizontal bow tie. (**c**) One month postoperatively, wound healing mechanisms have started replacing ablated tissue. This has reduced the spherical equivalent to +0.50D, and the corneal flattening is less marked. (**d**) By 1 year, the refraction has stabilised to −0.25D spherical equivalent, and the topography again appears less flat than previously

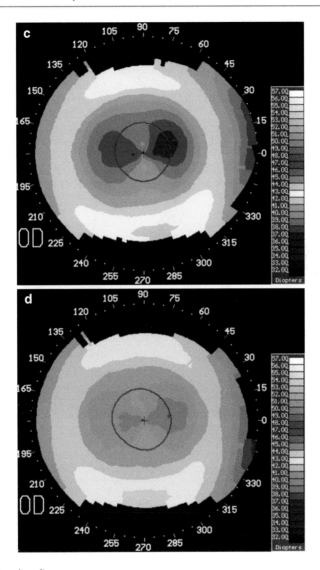

Fig. 14.1 (continued)

Regular Astigmatism

Regular astigmatism is corrected by the differential ablation of tissue in the steeper meridian, and therefore the treatment zone is usually hemicylindrical or oval (Fig. 14.5). As this involves the removal of tissue from part of the optical zone, a purely astigmatic correction is usually associated with some central corneal flattening and a corresponding hyperopic shift in the spherical equivalent [18]. The coupling seen following incisional procedures does not occur, because the middle and deep stromal lamellae are still intact. Astigmatic corrections are frequently performed in combination with spherical procedures [19].

Fig. 14.2 Photorefractive keratectomy (PRK) difference maps. The most effective way of displaying the change occurring is on a difference map. (**a**) The change induced by the surgery is obtained by subtracting the preoperative map (Fig. 14.1a) from the immediate postoperative map (Fig. 14.1b). The treatment zone appears blue because tissue was removed by the treatment. If the two maps are similarly aligned, there should be no change in the region outside the treatment zone. This is useful for medicolegally documenting the surgery which has been performed. (**b**) The change occurring postoperatively as a result of wound healing is obtained by subtracting a late map (Fig. 14.1d) from an immediate postoperative map (Fig. 14.1b). The treatment zone appears red because since the ablation, new tissue has been laid down and the cornea has become less flat

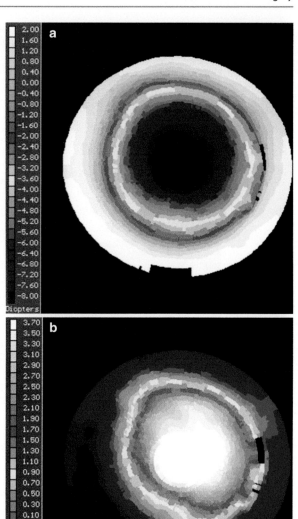

Irregular Astigmatism

Topography can be used to guide the excimer laser treatment of irregular astigmatism arising postoperatively or as a result of corneal disease. Originally in phototherapeutic keratectomy (PTK), fluid masking agents were used to protect depressions from the laser energy, whilst protuberances above the fluid level were ablated. This technique was useful for smoothing rough surfaces but lacked the precision required for a refractive procedure.

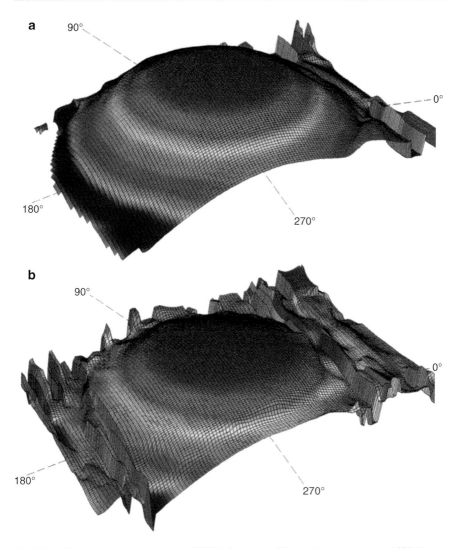

Fig. 14.3 Photorefractive keratectomy (PRK) height maps. This patient underwent −6.00D 6 mm PRK. (**a**) Three-dimensional representation of the preoperative corneal height. (**b**) Projection-based systems are able to accurately record the corneal topography immediately postoperatively. The central cornea has been flattened by the removal of the epithelium and ablation of the underlying stroma. The slightly heaped edge of the margin of the debrided epithelium can be seen just peripheral to the ablation zone. (**c**) The difference map shows the total depth of tissue removed by the procedure. For a myopic correction, more stroma is ablated from the centre of the treatment zone than from its periphery. (**d**) The cross section of the difference map shows the saucer-shaped ablation profile

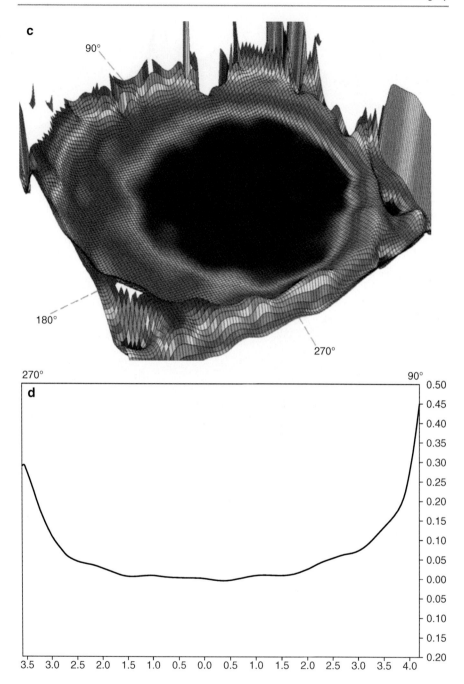

Fig. 14.3 (continued)

Fig. 14.4 Hyperopic photorefractive keratectomy (PRK). To correct hyperopia, the excimer laser removes an annulus of tissue from the midperiphery to steepen the central cornea. (**a**) Preoperatively, the cornea had a normal oval pattern. (**b**) One week after a +3.50D PRK, the refraction was −0.50D, and there was steepening of the central cornea. In the midperipheral cornea, the contours are closer together than normal, representing the rapid change from central steepening to flattening over the treated area. (**c**) By 1 year new wound healing tissue has been laid down where the ablation was deepest. This slightly reduced the effect of the correction, and the refraction stabilised at +0.25D

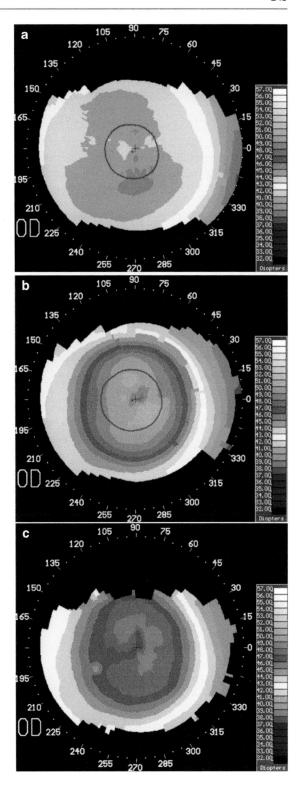

A few surgeons tried applying freehand small (e.g. 1 mm) treatment zones to patches of the cornea corresponding to the steep areas on videokeratoscopy maps. However, this commonly exacerbated visual problems by creating a multifocal cornea. Others have used Fourier techniques to better identify areas of irregularity by removing the spherical and cylindrical components of the corneal shape [20].

If topography is to be used to guide the correction of irregular astigmatism, it is imperative that height maps are used so that the treatment can be applied to the peaks, rather than the steep sides, of any elevated area. Ideally, the site and distribution of the ablation should be computer controlled, because any malposition of the

Fig. 14.5 Astigmatic photorefractive keratectomy (PRK). To correct astigmatism, the excimer laser removes more tissue in the steep axis than the flat axis. (**a**) Preoperatively the refraction was −3.00/−2.00 × 180°. The against-the-rule astigmatism appears as a horizontal bow tie. (**b**) One week postoperatively, the corneal surface is slightly irregular due to the healing epithelium. The overall pattern is almost spherical, although there is a very slight early overcorrection of the stigmatism centrally. (**c**) The difference map demonstrates that the power has been changed by approximately 2D in the vertical meridian and 5D in the horizontal meridian. (**d**) The height difference map shows that more tissue has been removed from the horizontal axis than the vertical axis and ablation appears oval

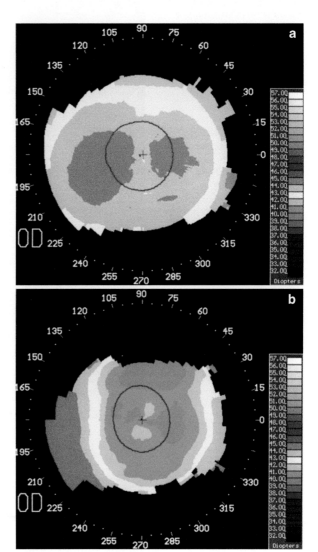

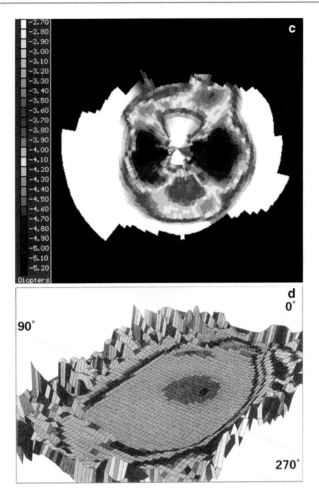

Fig. 14.5 (continued)

treatment can result in removal of tissue from the troughs rather than the peaks lead-ing to increased irregularity.

There are two potential mechanisms by which the application of laser energy could be controlled. Firstly, the topographic map could be used to lathe an indi-vidualised erodible mask complementary to the corneal shape, which was then correctly positioned in the path of the laser beam. Secondly, the topographic infor-mation could directly drive the ablation pattern of a "flying spot" laser, in which a computer-guided 1 mm beam is used to "paint" the corneal surface. Any of these techniques require that the subsequent wound healing is symmetrical. Even if they were able to smooth the surface of the cornea accurately [21], the refractive out-come would be difficult to predict, and the effect on visual function is currently unknown [22, 23].

Topography After PRK

As with any refractive procedure, the first postoperative map shows most accurately the topographic change achieved by the procedure itself. The treatment zone is usually easily delineated by the close proximity of adjacent contours at its edge. Its diameter can be measured using the grid or cursor facilities (Fig. 5.10). The position of the edge of the treatment zone is accentuated by the use of a difference map [24] (Figs. 14.2, 14.4c and 14.5c).

Myopic corrections result in flattening of the whole treatment zone (Figs. 14.1, 14.2 and 14.3). Following hyperopic corrections, there is steepening of the central cornea, which increases the corneal asphericity. This is surrounded by a ring of relative flattening at the edge of the treatment zone where most corneal tissue has been removed (Fig. 14.4). Sometimes this is not evident on the colour-coded contour map if a scale with a large step interval is used; but on the Placido image, the rings are more widely spaced in this region [16, 25].

For corneas that have round or oval topographic patterns preoperatively, the contours tend to remain concentric following spherical procedures. The appearance of a preoperative bow tie is changed little by a hyperopic procedure. However, following a myopic correction, the red bow tie is replaced by a blue bow tie in the perpendicular axis (Fig. 14.1). This arises from the way in which the corneal slope is measured by videokeratoscopes, and does not reflect a change in astigmatism.

In astigmatic procedures the treatment zone is oval. During the period of overcorrection, the preoperative red bow tie is replaced by a blue bow tie in the same axis (Fig. 14.5).

Following any PRK treatment, the induced flattening or steepening is most pronounced initially during the period of overcorrection and then becomes less marked with time as new wound healing tissue is produced (Fig. 14.1). This process and the subsequent remodelling may produce changes in the topographic pattern as described below.

In the early days of myopic PRK, small diameter ablations were used with the aim of minimising the volume of tissue removed. This resulted in wide individual variations in the refractive outcome. Some patients with a limited healing response were left hyperopic with persistent corneal flattening (Fig. 14.6). In contrast, those with an aggressive healing response underwent regression, with reduction of the corneal flattening and, in the worst cases, corneal steepening (Fig. 14.7). However, with the introduction of larger diameter ablations, cases of this severity are no longer seen [26, 27].

Projection-based topography systems are useful because they can measure the topography immediately postoperatively as they do not require the anterior corneal surface to be reflective [28] (Table 3.1). Height maps are particularly valuable for PRK because the refractive outcome achieved is directly related to the precise depth of tissue removed from the anterior corneal surface [15]. The difference between the preoperative and immediately postoperative maps demonstrates the profile of the ablation and the spatial uniformity of the laser beam. Subtraction of the immediate

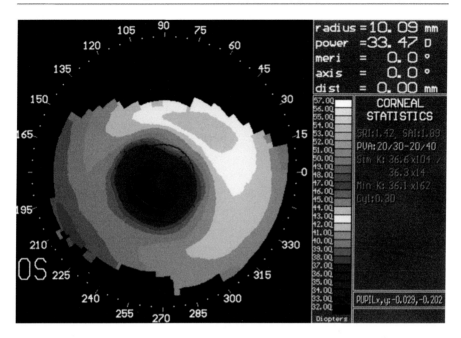

Fig. 14.6 Photorefractive keratectomy (PRK) overcorrection. Following a -6.00D 4mm PRK, the refraction in this 66-year-old man swung to +5.50D where it remained for about a year before slowly reducing to +5.00D over the subsequent year. He had extreme central corneal flattening (see cursor box) as a result of his minimal wound-healing response and never developed any haze. When wearing an optical correction, he suffered halos in moderate and dim illumination (Fig. 13.1). This was due to a combination of the small treatment diameter and the large +11.50 hyperopic shift. Fortunately such extreme cases are very rarely seen nowadays because larger diameter treatments are used

postoperative topography from subsequent maps quantifies the new tissue produced at intervals during the healing process [29].

Ablation Zone Centration

Accurate centration is best achieved by aligning the ablation on the centre of the pupil [30, 31], whilst the patient is fixating coaxially with the surgeon [32]. Alternatively, some surgeons fixate the eye by the use of a suction ring or other instruments, but this tends to be less effective [33]. Alignment is optimised by preoperative calibration of the aiming beams and the surgeon taking care to ensure that they are properly positioned on the eye before and during treatment.

Decentration most commonly occurs as a result of patient movement secondary to loss of fixation. The incidence is increased in higher-order corrections, presumably because the duration of the ablation is longer [34–37]. There is no correlation with the diameter of the ablation, but the visual effects of decentration are greater for smaller optical zones and in patients with big pupils (Fig. 14.8).

The risk of decentration can be reduced by the surgeon ensuring the careful preoperative counselling of patients to reduce anxiety, preoperative training of patients

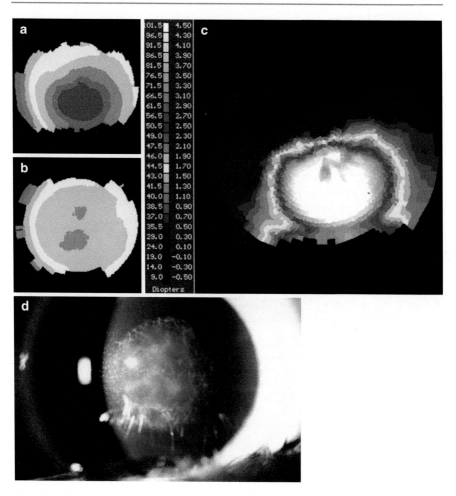

Fig. 14.7 Photorefractive keratectomy (PRK) regression and haze. Following a -6.00D 5mm PRK, there was an initial overcorrection of +2.25D, followed by a steady increase in regression until the residual spherical equivalent error was -7.00D at six months, when it stabilised. Subtraction of the one-year (**a**) from the preoperative (**b**) topography shows that the net result of the procedure has been a steepening of the cornea (**c**). This is due to an aggressive wound-healing response, which has produced excessive new tissue, causing severe corneal haze (**d**). Fortunately, cases of this severity are now very rare due to the use of larger diameter ablation zones

including fixation practice, comfort in the surgical chair, gentle support of the patient's head, vocal instructions and encouragement during the procedure [35, 38]. The surgeon should carefully monitor fixation throughout and stop ablating as soon as any movement occurs. The aiming beams can then be recentred and the procedure continued.

Differences in centration between surgeons are only partly explained by experience [39, 40]. This suggests that there may be variations not only in surgical skills but also in the ability of surgeons to make patients at ease. Technological advances

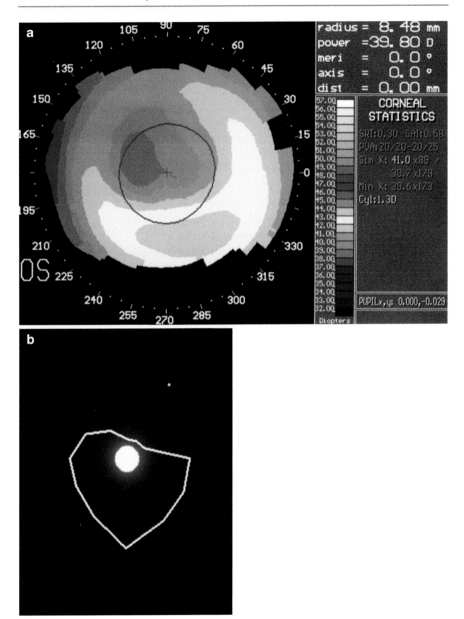

Fig. 14.8 Photorefractive keratectomy (PRK) decentration. A −5.25D 5 mm ablation zone was decentred superonasally by about 1 mm. (**a**) This resulted in marked asymmetry of the cornea (SAI = 0.58) and induced 2.00DC astigmatism. (**b**) The patient complained of halos below lights, and this was confirmed by objective testing. When viewing with his treated eye a bright central spot on a dark computer screen in a darkened room, he could trace the edge of his halo with the mouse cursor. The halo was most pronounced inferiorly because he has the equivalent of a very small diameter treatment zone in that area. The inferior cornea remains too steep, so the light passing through it defocused onto the superior retina, which is represented in the inferior visual field of the cortex (the inferior ray in Fig. 13.1)

aiming to improve centration during longer procedures include two types of eye-tracking systems [41]. The first automatically shuts off the laser when eye movement occurs. The second couples a real-time tracking device to mechanisms producing corresponding movements of the laser beam.

Decentration may be assessed postoperatively by using the software of the topographer to measure the distance from the centre of the flattened zone to the centre of the pupil (Fig. 5.10). In studies performed prior to the development of pupil detection software, measurements were made to the corneal reflex which located the corneal apex [30, 32, 42].

Measurements of decentration are best taken early after surgery, as soon as the epithelial irregularities have resolved, so the position of the ablation is not masked by asymmetric healing [43]. Ideally measurements should be taken immediately, but this requires a topography system which (unlike videokeratoscopes) can take measurements from non-reflective surfaces [28] (Table 3.1).

The results of published studies (Table 14.1) demonstrate that the magnitude of decentration has reduced over the years as laser technology and surgical experience has improved [39, 44]. Some authors have demonstrated no systematic error in the direction of displacement [39], whilst others have shown a tendency for decentration to occur either inferiorly [41, 45], inferonasally [35], superonasally [46] or down and to the right in both eyes [42]. The centre of the pupil shifts by as much as 0.4–0.7 mm at the extremes of miosis and mydriasis, but this occurs in a superonasal direction [47], and therefore preoperative miosis is not responsible for decentration. However, some surgeons have suggested that refractive surgical procedures should be centred on the natural pupil rather than one subjected to pharmacological constriction [35].

The topographic pattern resulting from decentration may be similar to that produced by pre-existing asymmetric astigmatism or an asymmetrical healing response. For example, a superior decentration may resemble a well-centred treatment performed in an eye with early keratoconus (Fig. 14.9). This highlights the importance of recording the topography preoperatively and as soon as possible postoperatively. These maps, and the difference map derived from them, may be the only way of determining the cause of subsequent irregular topography and whether the surgeon was responsible.

Table 14.1 Decentration of the ablation zone after PRK. A summary of tshe results of published work

Decentration	Mean (mm)	% ≤0.25 mm	% ≤0.50 mm	% ≤1.00 mm
Klyce and Smolek (1993) [145] phase IIA and B	0.79±0.11	10	13	52
	0.47±0.06	52	95	100
Cavanaugh et al. (1993) [168]	0.52		57	93
Cantera et al. (1993) [394]			75	95
Lin et al. (1993 and 1994) [462, 298]	0.34±0.23	37	85	98
	0.29±0.15			
Schwartz-Goldstein et al. (1995) [715]	0.46	22	65	97
Deitz et al. (1996) [845]	0.62±0.34		41	91

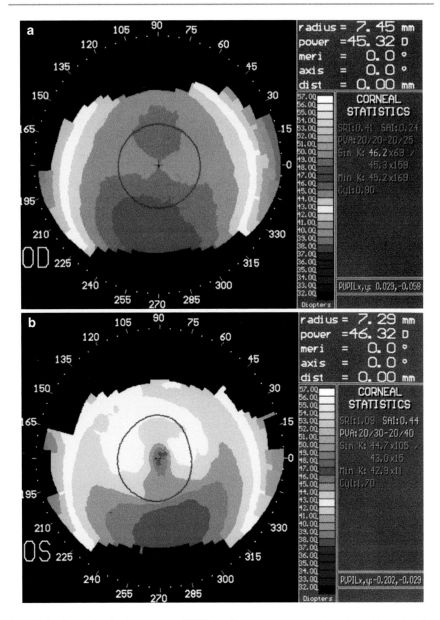

Fig. 14.9 Photorefractive keratectomy (PRK) in a keratoconus suspect. A patient with a refraction of −7.75/−0.75×180° underwent a left 5 mm PRK without corneal topography being performed preoperatively. After a large initial hyperopic shift (refraction about +4D at 1 week), he slowly regressed to approximately his original refraction (−8.00/−1.00×180°) with the development of grade 4 reticular haze. When topography was performed 15 months postoperatively, the left had the appearance of a superiorly decentred treatment zone. However, topography on the untreated right eye (**a**) revealed inferior corneal steepening which was compatible with a diagnosis or either a normal asymmetric bow tie or keratoconus suspect. The inferior steepening may have been more severe in the left eye (**b**) as this was the eye to be treated first. It is likely that the treatment zone was properly centred but that it was the pre-existing inferior steepening which made the topography appear decentred and gave rise to visual problems. An aggressive wound healing response with marked haze and regression is a recognised complication following the treatment of the eyes with keratoconus

The visual effects of decentration are determined by the diameter of the ablation zone and the size of the pupil. Early studies using small optical zones suggested that decentrations of 0.2–0.5 mm were clinically significant [30], whereas more recent studies using larger diameter treatments suggested that patients can tolerate up to 1 mm decentration [42]. The resultant irregular astigmatism can reduce visual acuity and contrast sensitivity. Patients may complain of polyopia and halos displaced in the opposite direction from the decentration (because the halo is largest where the radius of the treatment zone is smallest) (Fig. 14.8b).

Patterns of Healing

After PRK, new wound healing tissue is laid down over the surface of the ablation. The distribution of this new tissue determines the shape of the postoperative corneal surface. After surgery there is usually an increase in astigmatism and surface irregularity, which tends to improve with time [48, 49].

Eight corneal topographic patterns occurring after PRK have been identified (Table 14.2) [39, 44, 50, 51]. Patients with a homogeneous pattern have least astigmatism; and those with regular patterns (homogeneous or toric) have a better refractive predictability, visual acuity and level of satisfaction than those with irregular patterns [50]. The irregular patterns include semicircular (Fig. 14.10), keyhole (Fig. 14.11), central islands (Fig. 14.12), focal irregularities and irregularly irregular.

The incidence of different patterns varies between studies (Table 14.3). This may partly relate to the huge variation in healing patterns seen in different patients. In addition, it may also partly depend upon the characteristics of the laser, surgical technique and the topography system used. Surface irregularities are more likely to be detected by a device with a smaller central ring diameter and less smoothing in the algorithms, as in the TMS rather than the EyeSys.

Table 14.2 Topographic patterns after PRK [462, 298, 716]

Pattern	Description
Regular	
Homogeneous	Uniform flattening and smooth change of power, progressively decreasing power change towards periphery
Toric with axis	Smooth toric bow tie with greater induced flattening in the steep preoperative axis leading to a reduction in astigmatism
Toric against axis	Smooth toric bow tie with greater induced flattening in the flat preoperative axis, leading to an increase in astigmatism
Irregular	
Semicircular	General foreshortening of the ablation zone in one meridian
Keyhole	Area of relatively less flattening extending in from the periphery
Central island	Central area of relatively less flattening >1 mm in size and >1.00D in power
Focal variants	Generally homogeneous pattern with irregularities <1.0 mm in size or <1.00D in power
Irregularly irregular	Generalised irregularities over the treatment zone, not conforming to the specific criteria on any other pattern: more than one area >0.5 mm in size and >0.50D in power or one area >1.0 mm in size and >1.00D in power

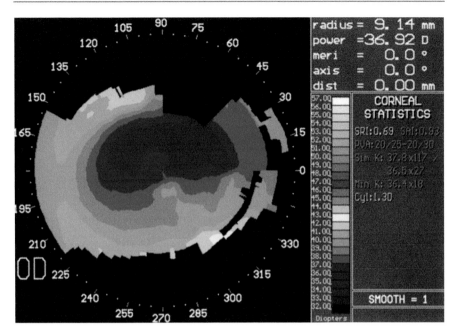

Fig. 14.10 Semicircular pattern (myopic PRK). One month following a −6.00D PRK, a greater quantity of new wound healing tissue has been generated inferiorly than superiorly, leading to asymmetry of the ablation zone. The best-corrected visual acuity is reduced to 6/9, the SAI is elevated, and the haze is denser inferiorly. The central topography became more regular during the following months

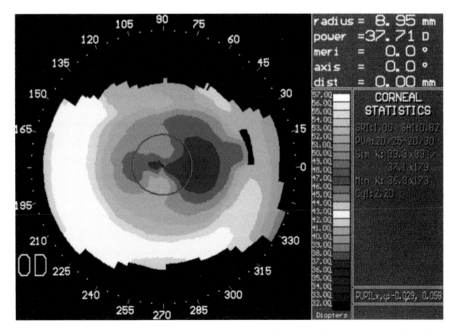

Fig. 14.11 Keyhole pattern (myopic PRK). One month after a −6.00D PRK, irregularity of the wound healing response has given rise to a keyhole topographic appearance

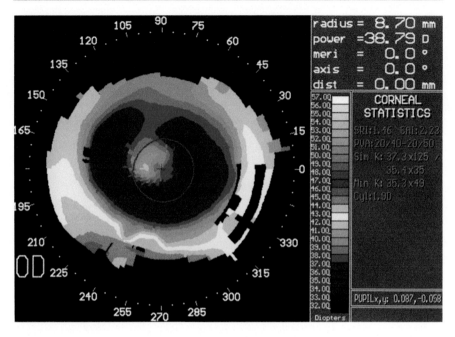

Fig. 14.12 Central island (myopic PRK). One week after a −3.00/−2.00 × 90° PRK, there is a central area of high power surrounded by an annulus of lesser power. Over the following months, the central island became less obvious, and the statistical indices reverted towards normal

Table 14.3 Incidence of topographic patterns after PRK [462, 298, 716, 982]

Lin et al. (1993 and 1994)			Hersh et al. (1995 and 1997)		
VISX laser			Summit laser, 4.5–5 and 6 mm		
TMS videokeratoscope			EyeSys videokeratoscope		
1 month postoperatively			1 year postoperatively		
Central uniform flat zone	45%	44%	*Homogeneous*	59%	21%
			Toric-with-axis-configuration	18%	28%
			Toric-against-axis configuration	3%	10%
Semicircular ablations	33%	18%	*Semicircular/keyhole pattern*	3%	25%
Keyhole patterns	12%	12%			
Central islands	10%	26%	*Central islands*	0%	0%
			Focal irregularities	4%	9%
			Irregularly irregular	13%	7%

Following astigmatic procedures, healing may be associated with a change in axis, the development of a homogeneous pattern if the astigmatism is corrected or reversion to the original axis. Irregular patterns may develop, similar to those seen following spherical procedures.

Central Islands

Central islands are a topographic complication of PRK that are relatively rarely seen since the early days of PRK [52]. However, they may still be evident in patients treated with early generation laser systems.

Table 14.4 Classification and incidence of central islands in patients treated with a VISX laser [52]. Central islands were seen in 67% of patients 3 months after surgery

Grade	Power	—	Diameter	Incidence
A	<3.00D			40%
B	>3.00D		<3 mm	14%
C	>3.00D		>3 mm	13%

Central islands are defined as any part of the treatment zone surrounded by areas of lesser curvature on more than 50% of its boundary (Fig. 14.12). They are classified according to the power and diameter of the central steep area (Table 14.4). No correlation was found with attempted correction [53]. The incidence and size of central islands are maximal soon after surgery and then reduce over time as corneal irregularities become smoother. In early studies, an incidence of 26% at 1 month was reported to reduce to 18% at 3 months, 8% at 6 months and 2% at 1 year [44, 54, 55].

Several mechanisms have been proposed to explain the occurrence of central islands [50–58]. Some of these mechanisms may also have a role in the determination of other postoperative corneal shape patterns. Each exerts its effects through one of the three common pathways: reduced central ablation due to characteristics of the laser, reduced central ablation due to properties of the cornea or irregularities of healing.

The difference in incidence of central islands between commercial makes of laser suggests that features of the individual lasers may be responsible. For example, ablations by Summit Excimer lasers are followed by fewer central islands than ablations by VISX excimer lasers. This may be because the Gaussian profile of the Summit beam removes relatively more central tissue than the VISX beam, which has a flat energy profile [57]. The variable incidence between different studies has led some authors to suggest that damage to the optical system of a laser can attenuate the beam, leading to "cold spots" where less energy reaches the cornea. It has also been suggested that the plume of effluent rising from the ablated surface could mask the beam [57, 58].

However, irregularities of ablation attributable to the laser should be detectable on preoperative laser beam analysis [59]. If this is not the case, differential ablation may occur as a result of mechanisms occurring in the cornea. It is known that the effective depth of ablation is determined by the hydration of the cornea: the greater the hydration of the cornea, the less corneal tissue is removed with each pulse. In theory, central islands could occur as a result of greater hydration of the central or deeper portions of the cornea [44], but there is little evidence to support this. An alternative theory suggests that, as opposed to differential hydration occurring naturally, "shock waves" produced by a flat beam profile "push" fluid centrally. However, experimental evidence of this occurring is lacking.

The great variation between individuals in the shape of the postoperative surface is more characteristic of a biological explanation. A slight irregularity and heaping of the epithelium is commonly seen at the site of closure of healing epithelial defects, including those following PRK. Normally this becomes smooth fairly rapidly, but persistence could account for some central islands. When epithelial heaping over a small stromal defect occurs, it may be incorporated into the epithelial thickening that is frequently seen. However, when the stromal defect is larger, the heaping may be surrounded by an area of relatively normal epithelium, and therefore it may become identifiable as an isolated island. This may account for the greater incidence of central islands in larger diameter ablations.

Central islands are more likely to be epithelial than subepithelial, because they are seldom associated with a localised increase in corneal haze. However, subepithelial changes may be responsible for the asymmetric or semicircular appearance of some ablations, where a wedge of increased haze is associated with relative corneal steepening and foreshortening of the ablation zone.

In any group of patients with irregularity of the postoperative corneal surface, there are probably several different mechanisms acting, either alone or in combination in different patients. The prevention of irregularities therefore requires a combined approach. Some surgeons have applied more pulses to the central 2–3 mm of the cornea, either by manually performing a shallow PTK beforehand, or by using laser algorithms with an automatic correction [57], or as a second procedure [60]. In addition, it should also be possible to modify the ablation profile to favour regular wound healing.

Long-Term Follow-Up

It has been shown that the anterior corneal topography continues to change up to 14 years post-treatment [61]. Studies have reported a mean regression of −0.5 dioptres over the first 1–2 years with a slow continued myopic regression over the following 12–14 years. However, most studies have assessed stability based on refraction and mean K readings which do not take into account various parameters including the posterior corneal surface and normal age-related changes in the cornea, lens and vitreous [61].

Laser In Situ Keratomileusis

The use of the excimer laser in refractive surgery has overcome the variability of surgical technique characteristic of incisional procedures. However, suboptimal accuracy, predictability and stability of the refractive change still persist following PRK due to variability of the wound healing response. In recent years, laser in situ keratomileusis (LASIK) has been introduced with the aim of controlling wound healing.

Mechanisms

LASIK was preceded by first manual, and then automated, keratomileusis or lamellar keratoplasty [62]. In these procedures the anterior corneal surface was reshaped by cutting the superficial tissues. LASIK is more refined and involves creating a corneal flap with a microkeratome or femtosecond laser, ablating the stromal bed with an excimer laser to produce the refractive correction and then replacing the flap [63]. The flap is usually 120–190 μm thick and 7.2–8.5 mm in diameter, with a 1 mm hinge. At least 30% of the corneal thickness should remain undisturbed to avoid possible subsequent ectasia [64]. In contrast to PRK, the stromal wound can heal without the influence of the epithelium, and this results in less corneal haze.

Femtosecond Laser

Femtosecond laser is infrared with a wavelength of 1053 nm, and it produces photodisruption or photoionization of the corneal tissue in a similar manner to Nd:YAG laser. It generates a rapidly expanding cloud of electrons and ionised molecules, and the acoustic shock wave disrupts the treated tissue 2. A Nd:YAG laser has a nanosecond pulse duration (10^{-9} s), whereas femtosecond laser pulse duration is in the femtosecond range (10^{-15} s). Reducing the pulse duration reduces the amount of collateral tissue damage making it safer for corneal refractive procedures.

Topography After LASIK

The refractive and topographic changes after LASIK are similar to PRK, with an initial overcorrection being followed by a gradual return towards emmetropia [65, 66]. However, because the surface epithelium remains intact, videokeratoscopy can be performed successfully at an earlier stage, and the corneal surface is regular within days [67]. Some authors suggest that the overcorrection is not as large and that stability is reached at an earlier stage [65, 67].

Significant decentration (>0.5 mm) occurs in 16–50% of patients undergoing LASIK [45, 64, 66]. Its frequency and severity is up to twice that of PRK [45]. This may partly arise because the stromal bed is more difficult to mark than the epithelium. In addition, the higher-order corrections typically treated by LASIK are associated with, firstly, longer treatment times during which drift may occur and, secondly, difficulty seeing the fixation target due to worse unaided vision and the greater ablation depth.

Despite the ablation being covered by a flap of corneal tissue, surface irregularities may occur [62, 65]. Central islands are similar to those seen after PRK [64–66]. In the past, suturing of the flap could contribute to irregularities, but now most surgeons float the flap on fluid until it reaches its natural resting place as determined by the hinge and then rely upon drying to hold the flap in place without sutures [66]. Irregularities may be caused by the particulate debris in the interface which can be seen on biomicroscopic examination [64]. This is possibly derived from defective cellulose sponges, the microkeratome blade, the keratotomy incision or epithelial cells from the conjunctiva or lid margins swept onto interface by excessive irrigation or patient tearing. The feint punctate grey spots seen in the stromal bed of some patients are thought to be deposits of extracellular matrix material produced during wound healing [65].

About 4–10% of patients develop surface irregularity as a result of epithelial ingrowth at the periphery of the flap-stromal interface. In the majority this is a

1–2 mm band confined to less than 120° of the circumference of the flap [66]. The most common sites are inferiorly and temporally. However, in some patients the epithelial front actively progresses across the cornea under the flap [64]. This causes increasing irregular astigmatism which reduces best-corrected visual acuity. Relifting of the flap and removal of the cells immediately restore the corneal topography and visual acuity (Fig. 14.13). Epithelial ingrowth is a risk factor for melting or necrosis of the corneal flap, so when severe, debridement should be performed early [66].

Fig. 14.13 LASIK epithelial ingrowth. A patient underwent a right −8.00D (79 μ) LASIK ablation under a 160 micron flap. (**a**) At 1 month the vision was only 6/24. On biomicroscopy there was a focal cystic lesion originating from the extreme periphery of the flap-stromal bed interface. Topography showed generalised flattening of the treatment zone, with localised steepening relating to the abnormality of the interface. (**b**) By 3 months it had enlarged and progressed across the cornea sufficiently to cause 4.00DC irregular astigmatism and reduce the best-corrected visual acuity to 6/18. (**c**) Four months after the original procedure, the flap was relifted, and the ingrowing epithelial cells were removed. This immediately improved the best-corrected acuity and restored the flattening across the whole ablation zone (Courtesy of Mr. Patrick Condon FRCS FRCOphth)

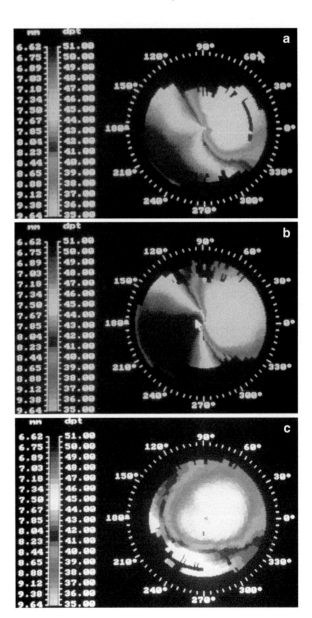

Small Incision Lenticule Extraction (SMILE)

Small incision lenticule extraction (SMILE) involves the cutting of a small intra-stromal lenticule using a femtosecond laser and its manual removal. It evolved from femtosecond lenticule extraction (FLEx), which allowed the removal of a stromal lenticule without the creation of a flap [67]. It is used to treat myopia, hyperopia, presbyopia and astigmatism and has been shown to have similar outcomes to LASIK [68].

As the anterior corneal stroma is preserved, it is thought that the corneal biomechanics are less disrupted compared to post-LASIK treatment: it promises similar clinical outcomes to LASIK with potential maintenance of biomechanical integrity [69–72].

Topography After SMILE

Topography patterns following SMILE are similar to those following LASIK as similar patterns of tissue are removed in both myopic and hyperopic treatments [73–74].

Complications

Complications following SMILE are rare and include epithelial abrasions, perforated caps, stromal keratitis and postsurgical ectasia. There have been numerous studies on SMILE outcomes, but most have included small patient numbers and short follow-up [67, 74–76].

Surface or Interface Complications
Between 4 and 10% of patients may get stromal microstriae, but these have not been shown to have any clinical significance [67, 76, 77].

Other problems include corneal haze, sterile inflammation, minor islands of interface epithelial cells and interface debris [78].

Ectasia Post-SMILE
Postoperative ectasia remains the most feared postoperative complication for any refractive surgeon. Whilst rare, it does still occur [79–83], but its occurrence should be minimised by a thorough preoperative assessment similar to that for LASIK.

Laser Thermal Keratoplasty

Laser thermokeratoplasty is a surface technique which acts by structurally altering the tissues of the superficial cornea to change its anterior curvature [66, 84, 85].

Mechanisms

When collagen is heated to 50–55 °C, its interpeptide hydrogen bonds break, and the triple helical structure collapses. This results in contraction of collagen fibres to about one-third of their original length [85]. For over a century, this has been achieved using heated wires, thermal probes and radio-frequency or microwave probes. Recently the technique has been refined by the use of the infrared holmium:YAG laser (wavelength 2.1 μm) [66].

Topography After LTK

Each laser spot (diameter 300–600 μm) induces a cone of shrunken tissue, with its base on the corneal surface, and apex at a depth which increases with the total laser energy applied [10, 85]. This creates a flattened zone centred on the spot itself and a steepened zone surrounding it (Fig. 14.14b). The refractive effect achieved is dependent upon the location of the spots and their proximity to their neighbours [84].

The holmium:YAG laser utilises a polyprismatic lens to divide its beam into eight spots organised in a ring, which is centred on the pupil [66] (Fig. 14.14a). If the ring has a diameter of 3 mm or less, opposite spots are sufficiently close together that their central flattened zones overlap. This results in flattening of the optical zone of the cornea, which could theoretically be used for the treatment of myopia (Fig. 14.14c). In practice, the proximity of the altered corneal stroma to the visual axis limits its use in these cases.

At a ring diameter of 4 mm, the refractive effect is small and unpredictable because the flattened zones and steepened zones of opposite spots overlap (Fig. 14.14d).

When the diameter of the ring is 5 mm or greater, opposite spots are sufficiently far apart that the optical zone of the cornea is only steepened (Fig. 14.14e). This technique is practised for the treatment of hyperopia, when ring diameters of 6–8 mm are commonly used. Greater refractive effect is achieved by increasing the laser energy (energy per pulse or number of pulses) or the number of spots [86–88]. New spots can be added to the same ring between existing ones by rotating the delivery system through 22.5°, or a different ring diameter can be used. Postoperatively, the topographic maps show central steepening, with flattening of the corneal periphery (Figs. 14.15 and 14.16). Regression of effect is usually seen within 1 month and tends to stabilise after 3 months [86, 87].

Both myopic and hyperopic regular astigmatisms can be treated by selecting the appropriate ring diameter and then masking the spots in two opposite quadrants. When these treatments are applied experimentally to spherical corneas, the postoperative videokeratoscopy map demonstrates a blue or a red bow tie, respectively [84]. When used to treat astigmatism, a preoperative bow tie should be eliminated.

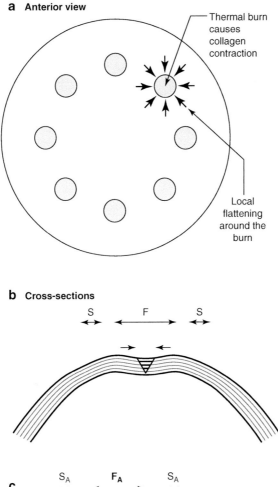

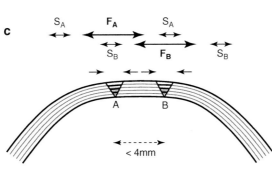

Fig. 14.14 LTK mechanism. The effect of holmium LTK on corneal topography. (**a**) Thermal spots are applied in one or two rings concentric with the pupil. (**b**) Thermal treatment has greatest effect superficially and therefore produces a cone of collagen contraction (thick black lines). This shortens the arc length of the superficial cornea (arrows) producing a flattened zone (f) centred on the spot itself. As a result the surrounding cornea is steepened (S). (**c**) When the opposite spots (**a** and **b**) are close together, the flattened zones overlap, resulting in flattening of the central cornea. (**d**) When the spots are 4 mm apart, the flattened and steepened zones overlap, producing a small unpredictable change in topography. (**e**) When opposite spots are further apart, the central cornea is steepened

Fig. 14.14 (continued)

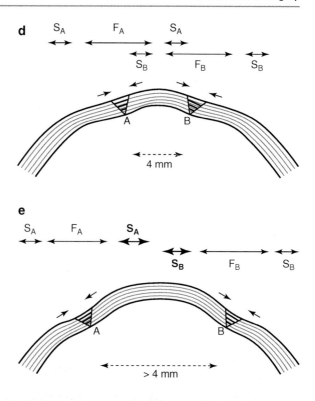

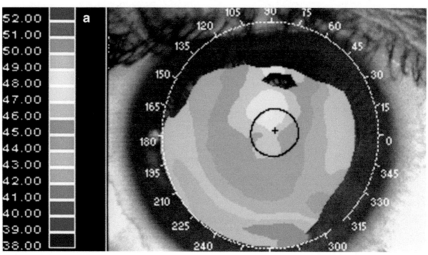

Fig. 14.15 Holmium LTK. The preoperative (**a**) and 1-week postoperative (**b**) maps of a patient who underwent a +3.00D laser thermokeratoplasty. The procedure induced steepening of the central cornea, flattening of the periphery and a rapid change in contour of intermediate zone

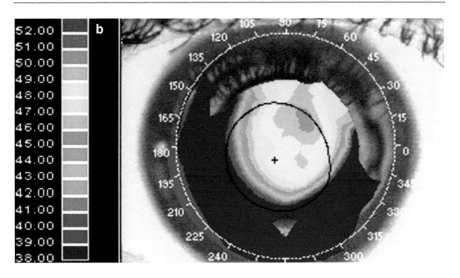

Fig. 14.15 (continued)

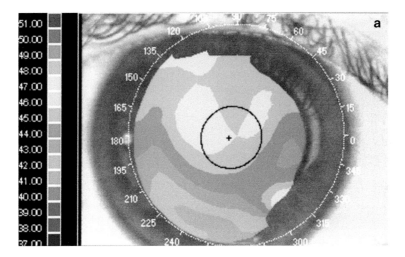

Fig. 14.16 Holmium LTK-induced change. In a patient with pre-existing against-the-rule astigmatism following cataract extraction, the difference between the preoperative (**a**) and 1-month postoperative (**b**) maps demonstrates that the +3.25D laser thermokeratoplasty induced a spherical change in the central corneal power (**c**)

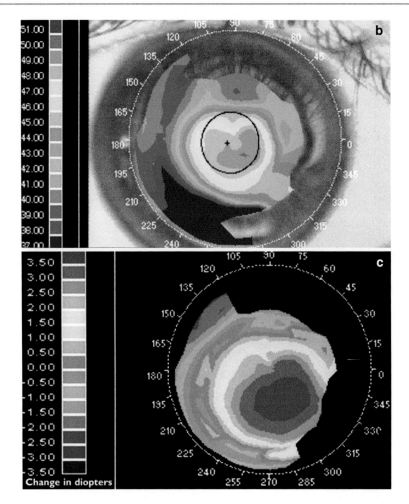

Fig. 14.16 (continued)

References

* References Particularly Worth Reading

1. Maguire LJ. Corneal topography of patients with excellent Snellen visual acuity after epikera-tophakia for aphakia. Am J Ophthalmol. 1990;109:162–7.
2. *Mandell RB. Corneal power correction factor for photorefractive keratectomy. J Cataract Refract Surg. 1994;10:125–8.
3. Thompson KP. Will the excimer laser resolve the unsolved problems with refractive surgery? [editorial]. Refract Corneal Surg. 1990;6:315–7.
4. Trokel SL, Srinivasan R, Braren B. Excimer laser surgery of the cornea. Am J Ophthalmol. 1983;96:710–5.

5. Marshall J, Trokel S, Rothery S, Krueger RR. Photoablative reprofiling of the cornea using an excimer laser: photorefractive keratectomy. Lasers Ophthalmol. 1986;1:21–48.

6. Marshall J, Trokel S, Rothery S, Schubert H. An ultrastructural study of corneal incisions induced by excimer laser at 193nm. Ophthalmology. 1985;92:749–58.

7. Puliafito CA, Steinert RF, Deutsch TF, Hillenkamp F, Dehm EJ, Adler CM. Excimer laser ablation of the cornea and lens. Ophthalmology. 1985;92:741–8.

8. Marshall J, Trokel S, Rothery S, Krueger RR. A comparative study of corneal incisions induced by diamond and steel knives and two ultraviolet radiations from an excimer laser. Br J Ophthalmol. 1986;70:482–501.

9. Aron Rosa DS, Boerner CF, Gross M, Timsit J-C, Delacour M, Bath PE. Wound healing following excimer laser radial keratotomy. J Cataract Refract Surg. 1988;14:173–9.

10. Binder PS. What we have learned about corneal wound healing from refractive surgery. Refract Corneal Surg. 1989;5:98–120.

11. Corbett MC, Marshall J. Corneal haze after excimer laser PRK: a review of aetiological mechanisms and treatment options. Lasers Light Ophthalmol. 1996;7:173–96.

12. Corbett MC, Prydal JI, Verma S, Oliver KM, Pande M, Marshall J. An in vivo investigation of the structures responsible for corneal haze after PRK, and their effect on visual function. Ophthalmology. 1996;103:1366–80.

13. Durrie DS, Lesher MP, Cavanaugh TB. Classification of variable clinical response after myopic photorefractive keratectomy. J Refract Surg. 1995;11:341–7.

14. Niles C, Culp B, Teal P. Excimer laser photorefractive keratectomy using an erodible mask to treat myopic astigmatism. J Cataract Refract Surg. 1996;22:436–40.

15. Munnerlyn CR, Koons SJ, Marshall J. Photorefractive keratectomy: a technique for laser refractive surgery. J Cataract Refract Surg. 1988;14:46–52.

16. *Dierick HG, Van Mellaert CE, Missotten L. Topography of rabbit corneas after photorefractive keratectomy for hyperopia using airborne rotational masks. J Refract Surg. 1996;12:774–82.

17. Danjoux J-P, Kalski RS, Cohen P, Lawless MA, Rogers C. Excimer laser photorefractive keratectomy for hyperopia. J Refract Surg. 1997;13:349–55.

18. *Dausch DGJ, Klein RJ, Schröder E, Niemczyk S. Photorefractive keratectomy for hyperopic and mixed astigmatism. J Refract Surg. 1996;12:684–692.

19. Alpins NA. New method of targeting vectors to treat astigmatism. J Cataract Refract Surg. 1997;23:65–75.

20. Olsen T, Dam-Johansen M, Beke T, Hjortdal JO. Evaluating surgically induced astigmatism by Fourier analysis of corneal topography data. J Cataract Refract Surg. 1996;22:318–23.

21. Liang F-Q, Geasey SD, del Cerro M, Aquavella JV. A new procedure for evaluating smoothness of corneal surface following 193nm excimer laser ablation. Refract Corneal Surg. 1992;8:459–65.

22. Fleming JF. Should refractive surgeons worry about corneal asphericity? Refract Corneal Surg. 1990;6:455–7.

23. Oliver KM, Hemenger RP, Corbett MC, O'Brart DPS, Verma S, Marshall J, Tomlinson A. Corneal optical aberrations induced by photorefractive keratectomy. J Refract Surg. 1997;13:246–54.

24. *Johnson DA, Haight DH, Kelly SE, Muller J, Swinger CA, Tostanoski J, Odrich MG. Reproducibility of videokeratographic digital subtraction maps after excimer laser photorefractive keratectomy. Ophthalmology. 1996;103:1392–8.

25. Jackson WB, Mintsioulis G, Agapitos PJ, Casson EJ. Excimer laser photorefractive keratectomy for low hyperopia: safety and efficacy. J Cataract Refract Surg. 1997;23:480–7.

26. O'Brart DPS, Corbett MC, Lohmann CP, Kerr Muir MG, Marshall J. The effects of ablation diameter on the outcome of excimer laser photorefractrive keratectomy (PRK): a prospective, randomised, double blind study. Arch Ophthalmol. 1995;113:438–43.

27. Corbett MC, Verma S, O'Brart DPS, Oliver KM, Heacock G, Marshall J. The effect of ablation profile on wound healing and visual performance one year after excimer laser PRK. Br J Ophthalmol. 1996;80:224–34.

28. Corbett MC, O'Brart DPS, Stultiens BAT, Jongsma FHM, Marshall J. Corneal topography using a new moiré image-based system. Eur J Implant Ref Surg. 1995;7:353–70.

29. Corbett MC, Oliver KM, Verma S, Pande M, Patel S, Marshall J. The contribution of the corneal epithelium to the refractive changes occurring after excimer laser PRK. Invest Ophthalmol Vis Sci (in press).
30. Uozato H, Guyton DL. Centring corneal surgical procedures. Am J Ophthalmol. 1987;103:264–75.
31. Guyton DL. More on optical zone centration [letter]. Ophthalmology. 1994;101:793.
32. Terrell J, Bechara SJ, Nesburn A, Waring GO, Macy J, Maloney RK. The effect of globe fixation on ablation zone centration in photorefractive keratectomy. Am J Ophthalmol. 1995;119:612–9.
33. Cantera E, Cantera I, Olivieri L. Corneal topographic analysis of photorefractive keratectomy in 175 myopic eyes. Refract Corneal Surg. 1993;9(Suppl):S19–22.
34. Schwartz-Goldstein BH, Hersh PS, The Summit Photorefractive Keratectomy Topography Study Group. Corneal topography of phase III excimer laser photorefractive keratectomy: optical zone centration analysis. Ophthalmology. 1995;102:951–62.
35. *Deitz MR, Piebenga LW, Matta CS, Tauber J, Anello RD, DeLuca MC. Ablation zone centration after photorefractive keratectomy and its effects on visual outcome. J Cataract Refract Surg. 1996;22:696–701.
36. Spadea L, Sabetti L, Balestrazzi E. Effect of centring excimer laser PRK on refractive results: a corneal topography study. Refract Corneal Surg. 1993;9(Suppl):S22–5.
37. Azar DT, Yeh PC. Corneal topographic decentration in photorefractive keratectomy: treatment displacement vs intraoperative drift. Am J Ophthalmol. 1997;124:312–20.
38. Klyce SD, Smolek MK. Corneal topography of excimer laser photorefractive keratectomy. J Cataract Refract Surg. 1993;19(Suppl):122–30.
39. Lin DTC, Sutton HF, Berman M. Corneal topography following excimer photorefractive keratectomy for myopia. J Cataract Refract Surg. 1993;19(Suppl):149–54.
40. Amano S, Tanaka S, Kimiya S. Topographical evaluation of centration of excimer laser myopic photorefractive keratectomy. J Cataract Refract Surg. 1994;20:616–9.
41. Maloney RK. Corneal topography and optical zone location in photorefractive keratectomy. Refract Corneal Surg. 1990;6:363–71.
42. *Cavanaugh TB, Durrie DS, Riedel SM, Hunkeler JD, Lesher MP. Topographical analysis of the centration of excimer laser photorefractive keratectomy. J Cataract Refract Surg. 1993;19(Suppl):136–43.
43. Sun R, Gimbel HV, DeBroff BM. Recommendation for correctly analyzing photorefractive keratectomy centration data. J Cataract Refract Surg. 1995;21:4–5.
44. *Lin DTC. Corneal topographic analysis after excimer laser photorefractive keratectomy. Ophthalmology. 1994;101:1423–39.
45. *Mulhern MG, Foley-Nolan A, O'Keefe M, Condon PI. Topographical analysis of ablation centration after excimer laser photorefractive keratectomy and laser in situ keratomileusis for high myopia. J Cataract Refract Surg. 1997;23:488–94.
46. Webber SK, McGhee CNJ, Bryce IG. Decentration of photorefractive keratectomy ablation zones after excimer laser surgery for myopia. J Cataract Refract Surg. 1996;22:299–303.
47. Fay AM, Trokel SL, Myers JA. Pupil diameter and the principal ray. J Cataract Refract Surg. 1992;18:348–51.
48. Cantera E, Cantera I, Olivieri L. Qualitative evaluation of photorefractive keratectomy with computer assisted corneal topography. J Refract Corneal Surg. 1994;10(Suppl):296–8.
49. Grimm B, Waring GO, Ibrahim O. Regional variation in corneal topography and wound healing following photorefractive keratectomy. J Refract Surg. 1995;11:348–57.
50. *Hersh PS, Schwartz-Goldstein BH, The Summit Photorefractive Keratectomy Topography Study Group. Corneal topography of phase III excimer laser photorefractive keratectomy: characterisation and clinical effects. Ophthalmology. 1995;102:963–78.
51. Hersh PS, Shah SI, Summit PRK Topography Study Group. Corneal topography of excimer laser photorefractive keratectomy using a 6-mm beam diameter. Ophthalmology. 1997;104:1333–42.
52. Hafezi F, Jankov M, Mrochen M, et al. Customized ablation algorithm for the treatment of steep central islands after refractive laser surgery. J Cataract Refract Surg. 2006;32:717–21.

53. *Levin S, Carson CA, Garrett SK, Taylor HR. Prevalence of central islands after excimer laser refractive surgery. J Cataract Refract Surg. 1995;21:21–6.
54. Krueger RR, Saedy NF, McDonnell PJ. Clinical analysis of steep central islands after excimer laser photorefractive keratectomy. Arch Ophthalmol. 1996;114:377–81.
55. McGhee CNJ, Bryce IG. Natural history of central topographic islands following excimer laser photorefractive keratectomy. J Cataract Refract Surg. 1996;22:1151–8.
56. *Krueger RR. Steep central islands: have we finally figured then out? J Refract Surg. 1997;13:215–8.
57. Shimmick JK, Telfair WB, Munnerlyn CR, Bartlett JD, Trokel SL. Corneal ablation profilometry and steep central islands. J Refract Surg. 1997;13:235–45.
58. Noack J, Tönnies R, Hohla K, Birngruber R, Vogel A. Influence of ablation plume dynamics on the formation of central islands in excimer laser photorefractive keratectomy. Ophthalmology. 1997;104:823–30.
59. Gottsch JD, Rencs EV, Cambier JL, Hall D, Azar DT, Stark WJ. Excimer laser calibration system. J Refract Surg. 1996;12:401–11.
60. Castillo A, Romero F, Martin-Valverde JA, Diaz-Valle D, Toledano N, Sayagues O. Management and treatment of steep central islands after excimer laser photorefractive keratectomy. J Refract Surg. 1996;12:715–20.
61. Lombardo M, Lombardo G, Ducoli P, Serrao S. Long-term changes of the anterior corneal topography after photorefractive keratectomy for myopia and myopic astigmatism. Invest Ophthalmol Vis Sci. 2011;52(9):6994–7000.
60. Helena MC, Robin JB, Wilson SE. Analysis of corneal topography after automated lamellar keratoplasty. Ophthalmology. 1997;104:950–5.
61. Pallikaris IG, Papatzanaki M, Siganos D, Tsilimbaris MK. A corneal flap technique for laser in situ keratomileusis: human studies. Arch Ophthalmol. 1991;145:1699–702.
62. *Condon PI, Mulhern M, Fulcher T, Foley-Nolan A, O'Keefe M. Laser intrastromal keratomileusis for high myopia and myopic astigmatism. Br J Ophthalmol. 1997;81:199–206.
63. Salah T, Waring GO, El Maghraby A, Moadel K, Grimm SB. Excimer laser in situ keratomileusis under a corneal flap for myopia of 2 to 20 diopters. Am J Ophthalmol. 1996;121:143–55.
64. Pérez-Santonja JJ, Bellot J, Claramonte P, Ismail MM, Alió JL. Laser in situ keratomileusis to correct high myopia. J Cataract Refract Surg. 1997;23:372–85.
65. Knorz MC, Liermann A, Seiberth V, Steiner H, Wiesinger B. Laser in situ keratomileusis to correct myopia of −6.00D to −29.00 diopters. J Refract Surg. 1996;12:575–84.
66. Parel J-M, Ing ETS-G, Ren Q, Simon G. Non-contact laser photothermal keratoplasty I: biophysical principles and laser beam delivery system. J Refract Corneal Surg. 1994;10:511–8.
67. Sekundo W, Kunert KS, Blum M. Small incision corneal refractive surgery using the small incision lenticule extraction (SMILE) procedure for the correction of myopia and myopic astigmatism: results of a 6 month prospective study. Br J Ophthalmol. 2011;95:335–9.
68. Reinstein DZ, Archer T, Gobbe M. Small incision lenticule extraction (SMILE) history, fundamentals of a new refractive surgery technique and clinical outcomes. Eye Vision. 2014;1:3.
69. Reinstein DZ, Archer TJ, Randleman JB. Mathematical model to compare the relative tensile strength of the cornea after PRK, LASIK and small incision lenticule extraction (SMILE). J Refract Surg. 2013;29:454–60.
70. Sinha Roy A, Dupps WJ Jr, Roberts CJ. Comparison of biomechanical effects of small-incision lenticule extraction and laser in situ keratomileusis: finite-element analysis. J Cataract Refract Surg. 2014;40:971–80.
71. Yang E, Roberts CJ, Mehta JS. A review of corneal biomechanics after LASIK and SMILE and the current methods of corneal biomechanical analysis. J Clin Exp Ophthalmol. 2015;6:6.. https://doi.org/10.4172/2155-9570.1000507
72. Dou R, Wang Y, Xu L, Wu D, Wu W, Li X. Comparison of corneal biomechanical characteristics after surface ablation refractive surgery and novel lamellar refractive surgery. Cornea. 2015 Nov;34(11):1441–6.

73. Ganesh S, Gupta R. Comparison of visual and refractive outcomes following femtosecond laser assisted LASIK with SMILE in patients with myopia or myopic astigmatism. J Refract Surg. 2014.; 2014;30(9):590–6.
74. Lin F, Xu Y, Yang Y. Comparison of the visual results after SMILE and femtosecond laser-assisted LASIK for myopia. Abstr J Refract Surg. 2014;30(4):248–54.
74. Shah R, Shah S, Sengupta S, et al. Results of small incision lenticule extraction: all-in-one femtosecond laser refractive surgery. J Cataract Refract Surg. 2011;37(1):127–37.
75. Hjortdal JØ, Vestergaard AH, Ivarsen A, et al. Predictors for the outcome of small-incision lenticule extraction for myopia. J Refract Surg. 2012;28(12):865–71.
76. Kamiya K, Shimizu K, Igarashi A, et al. Visual and refractive outcomes of femtosecond lenticule extraction and small-incision lenticule extraction for myopia. Am J Ophthalmol. 2014;157(1):128–134.e2.
77. Kamiya K, Shimizu K, Igarashi A, Kobashi H, Sato N, Ishii R. Intraindividual comparison of changes in corneal biomechanical parameters after femtosecond lenticule extraction and small-incision lenticule extraction. JCRS. 2014;40(6):963–70.
78. Ivarsen A, Asp S, Hjortdal J. Safety and complications of more than 1500 small-incision lenticule extraction procedures. Ophthalmology. 2014;121(4):822–8.
79. Sachdev G, Sachdev MS, Sachdev R, Gupta H. Unilateral corneal ectasia following small-incision lenticule extraction. J Cataract Refract Surg. 2015;41:2014–8.
80. Mastropasqua L. Bilateral ectasia after femtosecond laser-assisted small-incision lenticule extraction. J Cataract Refract Surg. 2015;41:1338–9.
81. Wang Y, Cui C, Li Z, et al. Corneal ectasia 6.5 months after small-incision lenticule extraction. J Cataract Refract Surg. 2015;41:1100–6.
82. El-Naggar MT. Bilateral ectasia after femtosecond laser-assisted small-incision lenticule extraction. J Cataract Refract Surg. 2015;41:884–8.
83. Mattila JS, Holopainen JM. Bilateral ectasia after femtosecond laser-assisted small incision lenticule extraction (SMILE). J Refract Surg. 2016;32:497–500.
84. *Simon G, Ren Q, Parel J-M, Ing ETS-G. Non-contact laser photothermal keratoplasty II: refractive effects and treatment parameters in cadaver eyes. J Refract Corneal Surg. 1994;10:519–28.
85. Ren Q, Simon G, Parel J-M. Non-contact laser photothermal keratoplasty III: histological study in animal eyes. J Refract Corneal Surg. 1994;10:529–39.
86. *Kohnen T, Husain SE, Koch DD. Corneal topographic changes after noncontact holmium:YAG laser thermal keratoplasty to correct hyperopia. J Cataract Refract Surg. 1996;22:427–35.
87. Koch DD, Kohnen T, McDonnell PJ, Menefee RF, Berry MJ. Hyperopia correction by noncontact holmium:YAG laser thermokeratoplasty. Ophthalmology. 1996;103:1525–36.
88. Goggin M, Lavery F. Holmium laser thermokeratoplasty for the reversal of hyperopia after myopic photorefractive keratectomy. Br J Ophthalmol. 1997;81:541–3.

Ocular Surgery

15

Corneal topography can obviously be affected by disease processes (Chaps. 8, 9 and 10) and surgery (Chaps. 11, 12, 13 and 14) directly involving the cornea itself. Changes can also occur as a result of surgery to adjacent structures, although techniques usually aim to minimise this. The underlying mechanisms are similar in both situations (Tables 8.1, 11.1 and 15.1), so once the principles are understood, they can be applied to different surgical procedures to predict or explain the induced changes in topography.

Assessment of the corneal shape is rarely required in patients undergoing noncorneal surgery. However, in these cases, corneal topography can be valuable postoperatively in the investigation of unexplained visual deterioration and in the development of new surgical techniques.

In this chapter, examples of the topographic changes induced by three noncorneal surgical procedures will be outlined to demonstrate how the principles and mechanisms described in the previous chapters can be applied in different situations.

Glaucoma Surgery

Many patients undergoing trabeculectomy have excellent preoperative visual acuity. However, a number of studies have indicated that such surgery can alter corneal curvature and lead to a reduction in vision postoperatively [1–4]. As the surgery involves the limbus and anterior sclera, there are several potential mechanisms which can underlie these changes.

© Springer Nature Switzerland AG 2019
M. Corbett et al., *Corneal Topography*,
https://doi.org/10.1007/978-3-030-10696-6_15

Table 15.1 Mechanisms responsible for topographic changes following non-corneal ocular surgery

Mechanisms	Glaucoma surgery	Retinal surgery	Strabismus surgery
External forces	Tubes and reservoirs	Pressure by explant	Tension in muscles
Tear film	Bleb related	Conjunctival disruption	Conjunctival disruption
Corneal surface	Epithelial irregularity after antimetabolites	–	–
Corneal stroma	Cautery	–	? 2° to interruption of blood supply
Surgical incision	Scleral flap	–	–
Location			
Length			
Depth			
Architecture			
Surgical closure	Scleral flap	Sclerostomy sites	–
Alignment			
Suture bites			
Orientation			
Material			

The first four mechanisms are similar to those seen in corneal disease (Table 8.1), and the remaining two are seen following surgery (Table 11.1)

Topography After Trabeculectomy

Immediately after surgery, shallowing of the anterior chamber induces a myopic shift which resolves after about 3 weeks [2]. Keratometry tends to demonstrate a temporary mild increase in with-the-rule astigmatism (vertical steepening) [1, 2], although topography suggests that this is more severe and can persist beyond 1 year [3, 5].

Three types of topographic change have been described: superior steepening (48%, Fig. 15.1), superior flattening (17%, Fig. 15.2) and complex irregular changes (35%, Fig. 15.3) which include central steepening and central flattening [5]. When performing trabeculectomies, surgeons can minimise postoperative visual disturbance by attending to the manoeuvres which can alter the corneal topography.

Mechanisms
Most trabeculectomies are performed superiorly, under the upper lid. Excessive scleral cautery can cause collagen to contract in a similar manner to that described for holmium laser thermokeratoplasty (Fig. 14.13). This can result in localised peripheral flattening, particularly if cautery is applied to the limbus, and associated steepening of the paracentral cornea superiorly (Fig. 11.1b).

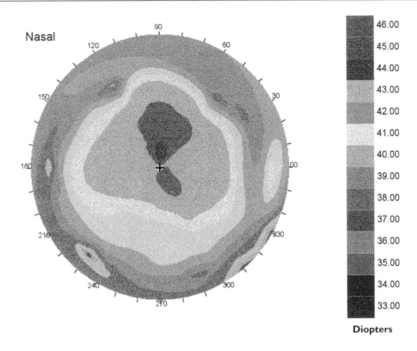

Fig. 15.1 Trabeculectomy steepening. Superior corneal steepening after trabeculectomy can result from two mechanisms. Excessive cautery can cause contraction of the scleral collagen fibres. Traction on the flap may occur if scleral sutures are too tight

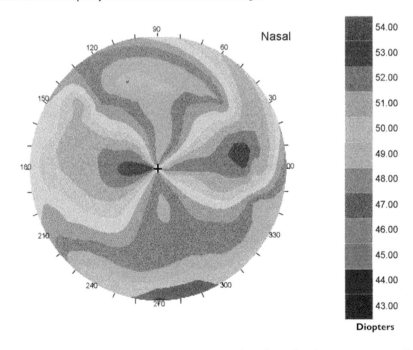

Fig. 15.2 Trabeculectomy flattening. Superior flattening after trabeculectomy can occur if the flap or the sclerostomy is made too large or sutured too loosely. In this case it was sufficiently severe to involve the central cornea and induce 5.00D asymmetric astigmatism

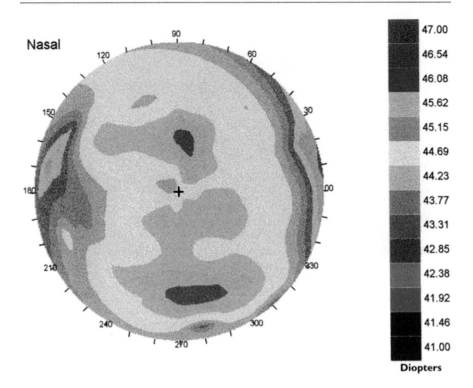

Fig. 15.3 Trabeculectomy irregular astigmatism. Complex irregular changes in the topography can occur if several factors are operating simultaneously. This case demonstrates a mixture of central flattening and superior torsion

When creating the scleral flap and the sclerostomy, the same principles apply as for incisions in corneal or cataract surgery. The topographic changes will increase with the size of the wound and its proximity to the cornea. It has been suggested that microtrabeculectomy is equally effective at lowering the intraocular pressure as the standard procedure [6], but it remains to be investigated whether the visual acuity and corneal topography would benefit.

Suturing the scleral flap too loosely or too tightly results in an increase or decrease in the arc length, and therefore radius of curvature, of the cornea. The effect is similar, although less marked, to that seen with corneal sutures (Fig. 11.1a, c). Likewise, dragging of the flap by uneven sutures can result in horizontal wound misalignment and irregular astigmatism (Figs. 11.1f and 15.4). If an absorbable suture is used, these effects can lessen over time.

If a large drainage bleb develops postoperatively, a meniscus of tear fluid can collect between the bleb and the cornea (Fig. 15.5). This causes localised peripheral flattening of the air-tear fluid interface in a manner similar to that seen with large pterygia (Fig. 8.8). The excessive use of antimetabolites such as 5-fluorouracil or mitomycin C, either intraoperatively or postoperatively, can cause epithelial

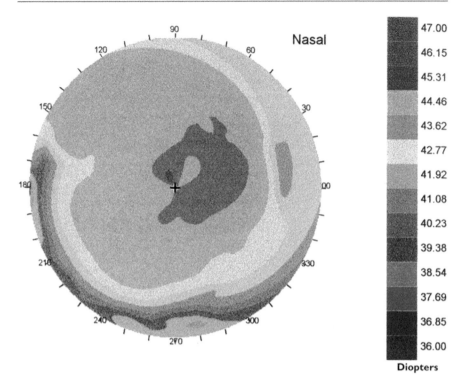

Fig. 15.4 Trabeculectomy misalignment. Malposition of the flap, causing it to be dragged to the left or right, results in torsional forces in the cornea and irregular astigmatism. As the flap is free on three sides, the effect of the sutures at its edge are transmitted through its base to the cornea

irregularity which is apparent on the corneal topography. Augmentation by the use of a drainage tube and subconjunctival reservoirs could theoretically produce local flattening with associated corneal steepening, but this is rarely seen.

Retinal Surgery

After posterior segment surgery, refractive causes of reduced acuity may be overlooked because full restoration of vision is not necessarily expected, as retinal malfunction is common. External approaches to retinal detachment repair involve the use of synthetic explants around the eye to apply pressure to the wall of the globe.

Topography After Retinal Surgery

Retinal detachment surgery involving explants commonly increases refractive astigmatism and may cause a myopic shift (Figs. 8.1 and 15.6) [7–12]. However, the

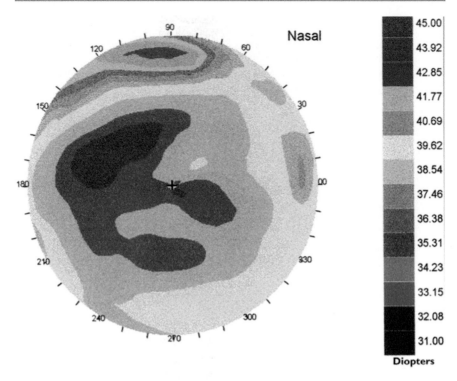

Fig. 15.5 Trabeculectomy bleb meniscus. This patient developed a large avascular cystic bleb after trabeculectomy augmented with mitomycin C. Postoperatively, the vision was good because the central cornea was regular. However, superiorly there was marked localised peripheral flattening produced by the tear film meniscus filling the angle between the bleb and the cornea (similar to the mechanism occurring in large pterygia; see Fig. 8.8)

refraction does not distinguish between alterations in corneal curvature and disturbances of other optical surfaces within the eye or axial length as aetiological factors. Long-term studies show that there is only moderate decay of the induced refractive astigmatism over 5 years, although it can be reversed by removal of the explant.

The topographic changes occurring after retinal detachment repair vary with the type of explant used. Local explants induce corneal steepening in the axis in which they are placed [1]. This is often asymmetric, with greatest steepening in the meridian nearest the explant forming an asymmetric bow tie. There may also be associated relative flattening in the perpendicular axis.

Of local explants, radial plombs induce greater corneal steepening than circumferential scleral buckles for three main reasons [10]. Firstly, they apply pressure over a more localised portion of the equatorial circumference of the globe. Secondly,

Fig. 15.6 Radial plomb. A superotemporal rhegmatogenous retinal detachment was repaired by suturing a radial plomb over the retinal hole just lateral to the superior rectus muscle. Preoperatively, the corneal topography showed a round pattern, but after surgery, the plomb had induced 2.00DC asymmetric astigmatism at 80°

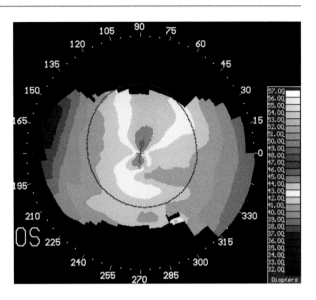

the plomb may extend more anteriorly towards the cornea because its position is not limited by the insertions of the rectus muscles. Thirdly, greater indentation may be achieved by a plomb made of compressible sponge than by a rigid silicone buckle.

When an encircling band is used, it is intended to generate an even pressure around the whole circumference of the globe. In cases where this occurs, peripheral corneal flattening surrounds an area of central steepening (Fig. 15.7). This commonly induces a myopic shift. A further contribution to this may be made by equatorial compression resulting in the elongation of the axial length. However, in other cases, the cornea appears quite asymmetric, with flattening on one side and steepening on the other. This may arise if the band is either sutured obliquely or tightened unequally [13]. The subsequent corneal distortion results in irregular astigmatism and a reduction in vision. It should be possible to avoid this complication by careful attention to surgical technique. However, it may be difficult to minimise other topographic changes without compromising the success of the procedure by limiting the height of the indent.

Mechanism

An explant causes flattening of the globe directly under the area of compression and steepening of the surrounding tissues (Fig. 8.1). Therefore an anteriorly placed explant may cause some localised peripheral corneal flattening as well as central steepening. Some more posteriorly placed explants may only produce a less marked corneal steepening.

Fig. 15.7 Encircling band. For more complex retinal detachments, an encircling band generates pressure around the circumference of the globe. (**a**) A tight band applying uniform pressure causes central corneal steepening and myopia. (**b**) When the band applies pressure unevenly, the cornea can become steep on one side and flat on the other

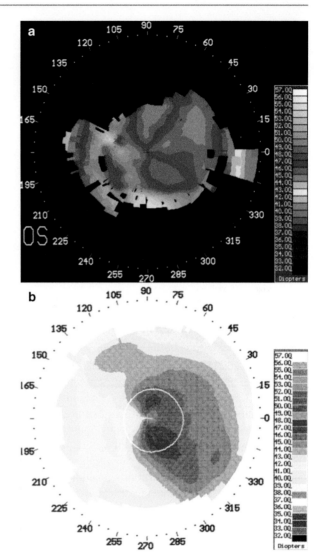

Vitreoretinal surgery and retinal detachment repair by an internal approach require a three-port vitrectomy. In this technique, short sclerotomies are made 3.5–4 mm behind the limbus. In theory, cautery and tight suturing at these sites could produce localised flattening, surrounded by an area of steepening which could extend to involve the cornea. However, this has not yet been studied, and nowadays, smaller sclerotomies are being used.

Retinal/vitreoretinal surgery can cause a significant increase in the corneal elevation and have a greater effect on the posterior corneal surface [14].

Any procedure which causes swelling and irregularity of the conjunctiva has the potential to disturb the tear film. This may cause pooling and meniscus formation (as described for pterygia and trabeculectomy blebs) or drying with dellen formation. The topography may be irregular or show localised flattening.

Strabismus Surgery

Squint surgery is often performed in children, in whom an uncorrected refractive error created by the procedure has the potential to cause or exacerbate amblyopia. Therefore it is important to use a technique with minimal effect on the corneal topography.

Topography After Strabismus Surgery

In patients undergoing strabismus surgery, as many as 60% have a small change in refractive astigmatism which quickly resolves [15, 16]. However, 2% of children and 25% of adults have an astigmatic shift of >1.00D which persists for over 1 year [17].

Refraction tends to suggest that those patients undergoing horizontal muscle surgery most commonly have a with-the-rule astigmatic shift (vertical steepening), whereas vertical muscle surgery is associated with an against-the-rule shift (vertical flattening). However, there is conflicting topographic data. Some studies have shown muscle recession to be associated with steepening [18], whereas others using animals have demonstrated it to be associated with flattening [19]. Further studies finding a lack of correlation between refraction and topography have supported a non-corneal aetiology for the refractive changes [20]. It has been suggested that extraocular muscle disinsertion might interrupt the vascular supply of the ciliary body and indirectly affect lenticular curvature.

Mechanism

It has been postulated that extraocular muscle tension plays a role in maintaining corneal shape. Theoretically, increased tension could flatten the peripheral cornea and steepen the central cornea, but it is difficult to predict the effect of muscles working in combination and how this would vary with the movement of the eye.

Topography could potentially be altered if the scleral suture bites are too large and tied too tightly, but the reattachment of muscles is usually sufficiently far posteriorly to avoid corneal distortion. Conjunctival swelling or disruption can cause tear film irregularity in a similar manner to that seen following retinal surgery. It has not been determined whether any of these mechanisms are clinically significant in strabismus surgery.

References

*References Particularly Worth Reading

1. Hugkulstone CE. Changes in keratometry following trabeculectomy. Br J Ophthalmol. 1991;75:217–8.
2. Cunliffe IA, Dapling RB, West J, Longstaff S. A prospective study examining the changes in factors that affect visual acuity following trabeculectomy. Eye. 1992;6:618–22.
3. Rosen WJ, Mannis MJ, Brandt JD. The effect of trabeculectomy on corneal topography. Ophthalmic Surg. 1992;23:395–8.
4. Chan HHL, Kong YXG. Glaucoma surgery and induced astigmatism: a systematic review. Eye Vision. 2017;4:27. https://doi.org/10.1186/s40662-017-0090-x.
5. *Claridge KG, Galbraith JK, Karmel V, Bates AK. The effect of trabeculectomy on refraction, keratometry and corneal topography. Eye 1995; 9: 292–298.
6. Vernon SA, Spencer AF. Intraocular pressure control following microtrabeculectomy. Eye. 1995;9:299–303.
7. Givner I, Karlin D. Alterations in refraction and their clinical significance. Eye Ear Nose Throat Monthly. 1958;37:676–8.
8. Jacklin HN. Refraction changes after surgical treatment for retinal detachment. South Med J. 1971;64:148–50.
9. Foire JV Jr, Newton JC. Anterior segment changes following the scleral buckling procedure. Arch Ophthalmol. 1970;86:284–7.
10. Goel R, Crewdson J, Chignell AH. Astigmatism following retinal detachment surgery. Br J Ophthalmol. 1983;67:327–9.
11. Weinberger D, et al. Corneal topographic changes after retinal and vitreous surgery. Ophthalmology. 1999;106(8):1521–4.
12. Ornek K, Yalçindag FN, Kanpolat A, et al. Corneal topographic changes after retinal detachment surgery. Cornea. 2002;21(8):803–6.
13. *Hayashi H, Hayashi K, Nakao F, Hayashi F. Corneal shape changes after scleral buckling surgery. Ophthalmology 1997; 104: 831–837.
14. Sinha R, Sharma N, Verma L, et al. Corneal topographic changes following retinal surgery. BMC Ophthalmol. 2004;4:10. https://doi.org/10.1186/1471-2415-4-10.
15. Marshall D. Changes in refraction following operation for strabismus. Arch Ophthalmol. 1936;15:1020–31.
16. Thompson WE, Reinecke RD. The changes in refractive status following routine strabismus surgery. J Pediatr Ophthalmol Strabismus. 1980;17:372–4.
17. Fix A, Baker JD. Refractive changes following strabismus surgery. Am Orthoptic J. 1985;35:59–62.
18. *Kwitko S, Feldon S, McDonnell PJ. Corneal topographic changes following strabismus surgery. Cornea 1992; 11: 36–40.
19. *Kwitko S, Sawusch MR, McKonnell PJ, Gritz DC, Moreira H, Evensen D. Effect of extraocular muscle surgery on corneal topography. Arch Ophthalmol 1991; 109: 873–878.
20. Preslan MW, Cilffi G, Yuan-I M. Refractive error following strabismus surgery. J Pediatr Ophthalmol Strabismus. 1992;29:300–4.

Index

© Springer Nature Switzerland AG 2019
M. Corbett et al., *Corneal Topography*,
https://doi.org/10.1007/978-3-030-10696-6

Printed by Printforce, the Netherlands